This book is a Gift 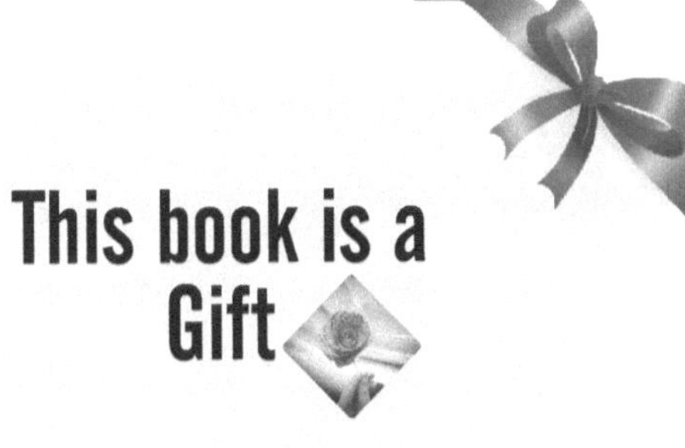

from

....

to

....

on the occasion of

....

date

....

"This book will reshape every woman's thinking, remold every woman's destiny, and drive them to the place of prayer."

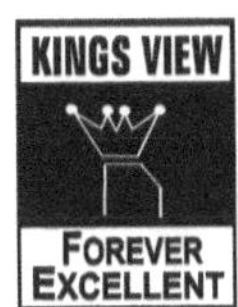

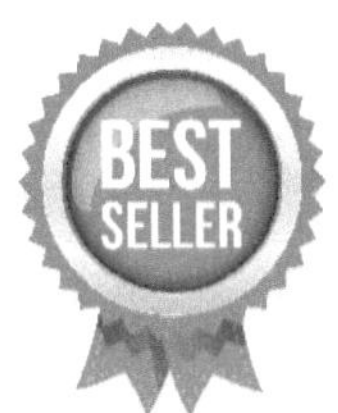

The Ministry of the WOMB

Fulfilling God's Creative Mandate for the Womb

"This book isn't only well-researched but also carries an unction for the transformation and re-arrangement of every woman's future and destiny."

INCLUDES OVER 50 DESTINY-TRANSFORMING LETHAL PRAYERS

the Ministry of the Womb

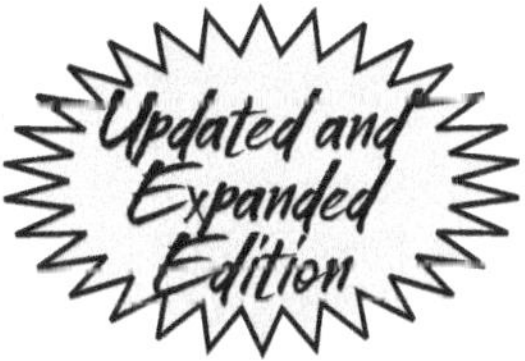

Augusta Ogbene

THE MINISTRY OF THE WOMB

First Edition - 2015
International Edition - 2021

Copyright © 2021 by **Dr. Augusta Ogbene**

ISBN: 979-848-75003-2-8

Published by:

KINGS VIEW PUBLISHING HOUSE
Calabar, Nigeria/ Tbilisi, Georgia
www.kingsviewbooks.com
E-mail: enquiries@kingsviewbooks.com
+995 568 286 737; +2347035358454

All Scripture quotations are taken from the Authorised King James version and The New King James Version of The Holy Bible, except otherwise indicated.

For further information, please contact:

Dr. Augusta Ogbene
Christian Women Intercessors for all Nations
Asaba, Delta State,Nigeria
www.cwifan.org
E-mail: cwintercessors@yahoo.com
+234(0)8036769278

Printed in the United States of America

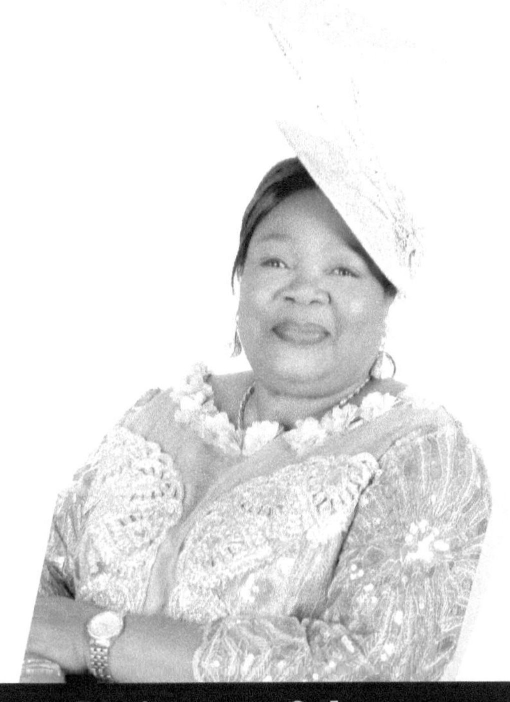

"*That our sons may be as plants grown up in their youth; that our daughters may be as corner stones, polished after the similitude of a palace:*"

Psalms 144:12

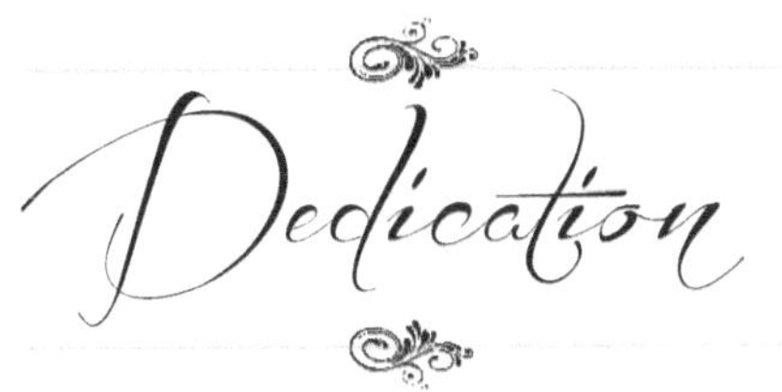

Dedication

I dedicate this book to

Women All Over the World

who yearn to honour God with their bodies and
fulfill the Divine mandate for their womb.

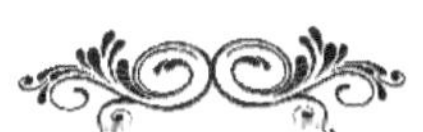

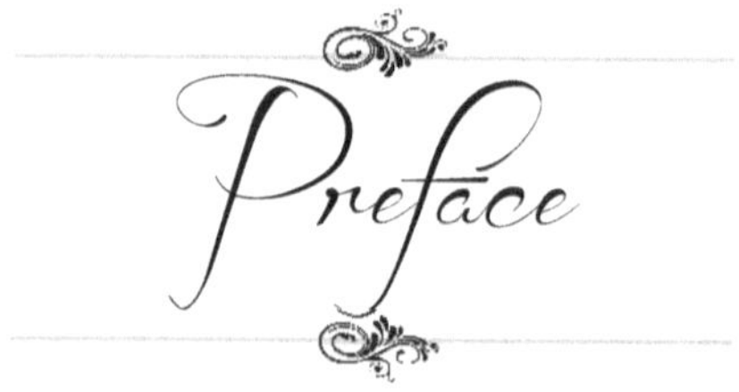 Preface

TO THE INTERNATIONAL EDITION

*Before I formed thee in the belly I knew thee;
and before thou camest forth out of the
womb I sanctified thee, and I ordained thee
a prophet unto the nations.*

Jeremiah 1:5

One of the greatest concerns of expectant parents relates to the physical and emotional health of their fetus. Yet, only a few parents seem to understand that this extremely important part of their child's life is shaped by the parents' environment.

Most parents are typically ignorant of the fact that a mother's emotional feeling during pregnancy can be transferred directly to her unborn child; her constant negative emotions can have a damaging effect on the fetus. This implies that a child's physical and emotional health is being shaped before it is even born.

But this isn't all about mothers. Latest studies indicate that how a man feels about his wife and unborn child is one of the single most important factors in determining the success of a pregnancy. A child hears his father's voice in the uterus, and there is solid evidence that hearing that voice makes a big emotional difference.

This book deals with deep mysteries surrounding the womb and the products of conception. It is an exposé on the untapped powers of a woman's womb and how it affects the unborn child. Each chapter unveils revelations and truths meant to reposition every woman to birth generational giants and champions.

Chapter one explains foundational issues

relating to the womb, as well as the physical and spiritual significance of the womb.

Chapter two focuses on the power of the womb; a deep revelation on the womb as the centre of every woman's power and creativity, and a place where women hold their stories and give birth to their visions.

Chapter three is an exposé on the womb as an altar - the meeting point of covenant between God and the unborn child; a mystery which will help every woman to understand why, like every other altar, the womb should be accepted and treated as sacred.

Chapter four provides a depth of explanation bordering on how the future of the unborn child is shaped from the womb. It relates, perhaps, to the most important occurrence in the life of a pregnant woman: Shaping the attitudes and expectations of her unborn child.

Chapter five is a detailed description of the original mandate of the womb from creation.

God created the womb with a specific mandate. What is this mandate? What is required of every woman to fulfill this mandate?

Chapter six opens up on the womb as a major gateway into a woman's spirit. Most of the things that have affected women all over the world were introduced into their lives through the gateway of the womb.

Chapter seven is a follow up to the gateway of the womb and focuses on polluted gateways. Once the gateway of the womb is defiled, the outcome or products of such wombs could be dangerously affected.

Chapter eight provides a complete recipe on rebuilding, revamping, and re-empowering the womb altar. It shows the way every woman can stand strong again, no matter how flat they had fallen.

Chapter nine unravels the mystery of birth defects from the womb. Why do most children suffer unnecessary defects? Why does God even have to allow it? What mystery lies behind this?

Chapter ten concludes this awesome treatise with a word on staying pure and unpolluted. That is, maintaining what God has done in your life and moving from glory to glory every passing day.

This book isn't only well-researched but also carries an unction for the transformation and re-arrangement of every woman's future and destiny. I believe it is a new day for this generation of mothers, and the generations to come.

Shalom!

Dr. Augusta Ogbene
Asaba, Nigeria

CONTENTS

Introduction

For so many years, lots of women have wrestled with several feminine challenges. Some of these include marital issues, scxuality, fertility, childbearing, and rearing.

Not many know about the Ministry of the Womb and how much it influences these feminine challenges. Some people's destinies have been altered by this ignorance.

On the other hand, people who have known and understood the mystery behind the Ministry of the Womb have had their lives changed.

This book is a thorough expose on the Ministry of the womb. It goes to show how the destinies of children and consequently, nations, are affected by the kind of womb that births them.

> **It is the lack of knowledge of the Ministry of the womb that has made some women give birth to human beings who have become a nuisance to their generation.**

Whoever a woman gives birth to (whether a president or a terrorist), most times, is a result of the consecration or desecration of her womb. In James 3:12 (GNT), a salient statement was made: "*A fig tree, my friends, cannot bear olives; a grape vine cannot bear figs, nor can a salty spring produce sweet water.*"

If the spirit in charge of a woman's womb is

that which works in the sons of disobedience, she will only give birth to a child subject to the operations of such a spirit.

On the other hand, if the Spirit of God rules over a woman's body and spirit, she will give birth to a child overshadowed by God's Spirit right from the womb.

Like begets like. It simply follows the law of nature. If the source is defiled, the product will be defiled. If the source is pure, the product will be pure and extraordinary.

From the foregoing then, it is apparent that the lifestyle of any child is determined right from the womb and his future is shaped ahead from there. For these to take place, there must be a bonding between the mother and the child in her womb.

But how can the lifestyle of the unborn really be determined from the womb?

How does the womb act as an altar for the bringing

of a new life into the world?

How does the pregnant woman bond with the foetus in her womb?

These are a few questions that this book answers in clear and helpful ways.

The book also shows that beyond overcoming the problems of barrenness and freely giving birth to children, God had a mandate for the womb, right from the beginning.

What is the mandate of the womb?

What should a woman do to fulfill God's original mandate of her womb?

These are all addressed in this book.

This book will reshape every woman's thinking, remold every woman's destiny and drive them to the place of prayer.

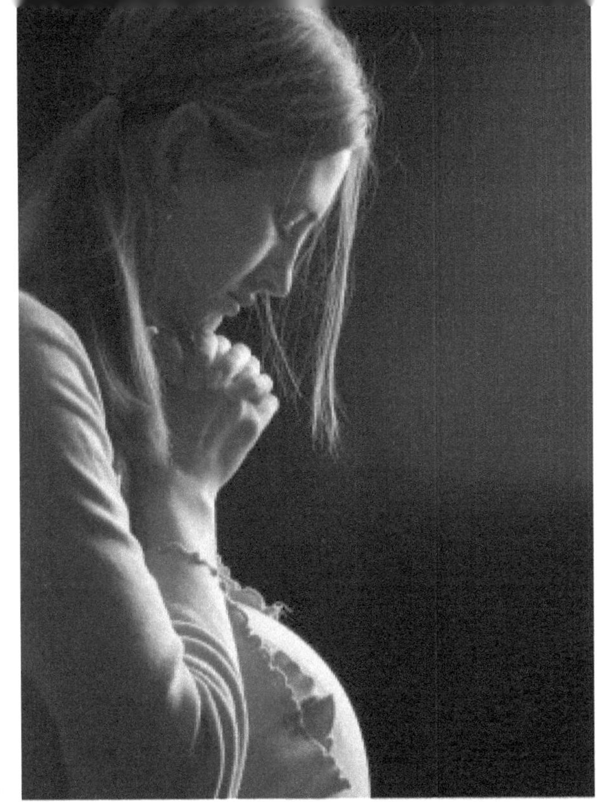

Chapter 1

THE FOUNDATION

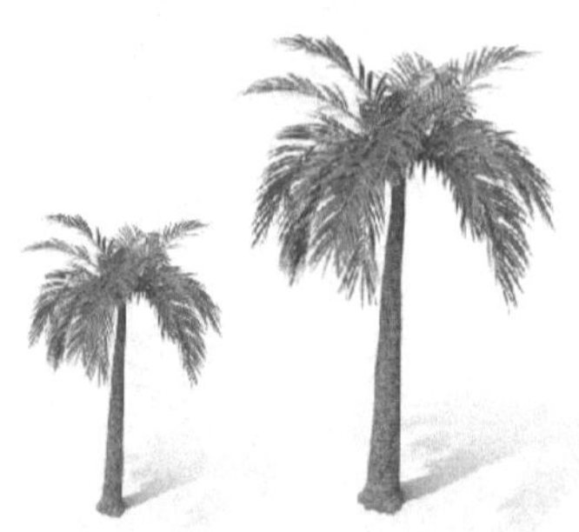

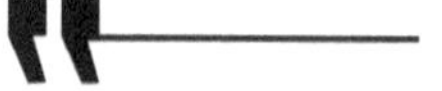
> *If the foundations be destroyed, what can the righteous do?*

Psalms 11:3

THE FOUNDATION

> " All women are life givers! They have the privilege of conceiving, nurturing, and bringing forth a miracle of life. "

What is a womb? A womb is an organ in the lower part of a woman's body part or female mammal where offsprings are conceived and in which they gestate before birth.

Actually, the womb is where the preparation

for the journey of life begins. The womb is the child's first home in life. Therefore, whatever happens in the womb, as the foundation of life, can positively or negatively influence an individual.

In any building project, the good construction of the foundation provides sustainable stability for the entire structure of the building. Once the foundation is faulty, the whole building will lack stability. This is probably the reason why the Scripture tells us that if the foundation is destroyed, the righteous have little or nothing to do to bring about a change.

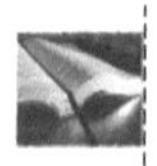 *If the foundations be destroyed, what can the righteous do?* **Psalm 11:3**

The womb, in a general sense, is a place of creation. It has the capacity to receive raw material and transform it into a finished product that can be admired by all men.

The womb can be likened to a warehouse

where destinies are kept or preserved. And using the woman's womb as a more natural explanation, we can say that,

the womb is a thing created or empowered by God to nurture or incubate a godly seed and give birth to a finished product after nine months.

The womb of a woman is a gift with many responsibilities. The following paragraphs throw more light on the physical and spiritual significance of the womb.

THE WOMB IS A WOMAN'S DISTINGUISHING IDENTITY

Webster explains that the word "woman" is a combination of the words, "womb" and "man."

"Woman," therefore, means "womb man" or "man with a womb." When God created the woman, He put within her a womb.

 *The Lord God caused a deep sleep to fall upon Adam, and he slept, and he took one of his ribs, and closed up the flesh instead thereof. And the rib, which the Lord God had taken from man, made he a woman, and brought her unto the man. And Adam said, This is now bone of my bones, and flesh of my flesh: she shall be called Woman, because she was taken out of man.* **Genesis 2:21-23**

THE WOMB IS LIFE GIVING

Genesis 3:20 (TLB) says, "*The man named his wife Eve, meaning, The Life Giving One!*"

Eve in Hebrew is *Chavvah* meaning, "Life Giver!" Eve was the prototype of all women - the first of her kind. She was a life giver.

All women are life-givers! They have the privilege of conceiving, nurturing, and bringing forth a miracle of life from within the womb.

Is it not sad that when women are meant to be "life-givers", many are rather "life-stoppers"? Examples are women who terminate unwanted pregnancies. These are life-stoppers.

▼

THE WOMB IS A BLESSING TO EVERY WOMAN

Genesis 49:25 (KJV) speaks of "*...the Almighty who shall bless thee with the blessings of the breasts and of the womb.*"

Every woman should receive her womb as a blessing from God. Before God gave conception and fruitfulness, He always blessed first.

Women need to affirm God's truth and confess that their womb is a blessing.

Before God spoke the words to Adam and Eve, "Be fruitful and multiply and replenish the earth," He first blessed them. God desires to bless every woman's womb. As a woman, you must pray for the health of your womb. Every husband should also endeavour to regularly pray over and bless the womb of his wife.

THE WOMB IS THE WOMAN'S GLORY

Hosea 9:11 (KJV) says, *"As for Ephraim, their glory shall fly away like a bird, from the birth, and from the womb, and from the conception."*

When Ephraim turned away from the Lord, God pronounced judgment upon them. His judgment was to take away their "glory."

What was their glory?

It was the conception of the womb.

Conception, pregnancy, and motherhood are the glory of a nation and it comes through the womb of women.

I declare God's blessing upon the womb of our daughters in Jesus' Name.

THE WOMB IS A HAVEN FOR MIRACLES

The greatest miracle in history took place in a womb! It was here that God became man! Jesus Himself was conceived in a womb! He identified with the womb of a woman.

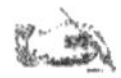

> *And the angel answered and said unto her, The Holy Ghost shall come upon thee, and the power of the Highest shall overshadow thee: therefore also that holy thing which shall be born of thee shall be called the Son of God. And when eight days were accomplished for the circumcising of the child, his name was called JESUS, which was so named of the angel before he was conceived in the womb.* **Luke 1:35; 2:21**

It is in the womb that miracles continue to

take place. Every child that is conceived in the womb is a miracle of God's creation. How blessed are women to have miracles take place in their bodies.

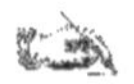

THE WOMB IS A SPHERE OF INFLUENCE

The Hebrew word *'rechem'* for womb is "matrix" which means "a place within which something originates or develops."

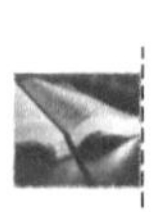

I the Lord your God am a jealous God, visiting the iniquity of the fathers upon the children to the third and fourth generation of those who hate me. **Exodus 20:5**

Iniquity is willfully following our own way rather than God's. Rebellion in parents can be passed on to children through the womb. Psalms 58:3 (KJV) says, *"The godless are perverse from the womb."*

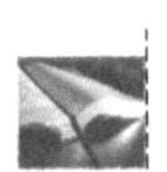

Yea, thou heardest not; yea, thou knewest not; yea, from that time that thine ear was not opened: for I knew that thou wouldest deal very treacherously, and wast called a transgressor from the womb. **Isaiah 48:8**

THE WOMB IS SACRED AND PRECIOUS, BUT CAN ALSO BE USED AS A PLACE OF JUDGMENT

Then David returned to bless his household. And Michal the daughter of Saul came out to meet David, and said, How glorious was the king of Israel today, who uncovered himself to day in the eyes of the handmaids of his servants, as one of the vain fellows shamelessly uncovereth himself! And David said unto Michal, It was before the LORD, which chose me before thy father, and before all his house, to appoint me ruler over the people of the LORD, over Israel: therefore will I play before the LORD. And I will yet be more vile than thus, and will be base in mine own sight: and of the maidservants which thou hast spoken of, of them shall I be had in honour. Therefore Michal the daughter of Saul had no child unto the day of her death. **2Samuel 6:20-23**

Michal received judgment upon her womb when she despised her husband and she died childless.

But it shall come to pass, if thou wilt not hearken unto the voice of the LORD thy God, to observe to do all his commandments and his statutes which I command thee this day; that all these curses shall come upon thee, and overtake thee: Cursed shall be the fruit of thy body, and the fruit of thy land, the increase of thy kine, and the flocks of thy sheep. And if ye walk contrary unto me, and will not hearken unto me; I will bring seven times more plagues upon you according to your sins. I will also send wild beasts among you, which shall rob you of your children, and destroy your cattle, and make you few in number; and your high ways shall be desolate. **Deuteronomy 28:15,18** and **Leviticus26:21,22**

Disobedience brought the curse of barrenness in these Scriptures. In Numbers 5:11-31, we read of how adultery brought judgment upon the womb. It says, *"the curse shall go into thy womb!"*

The womb should be kept pure. It should not be defiled through fornication or adultery. If this has been the case, there should be repentance, confession, and prayer for the cleansing of the womb.

The womb must be kept pure and holy for the nurturing of the "godly seed" that God desires.

The womb is a place where destiny can be enthroned or dethroned. For example, Esau's destiny as a firstborn was changed right from his mother's womb.

And the Lord said unto her, Two nations are in thy womb, and two manner of

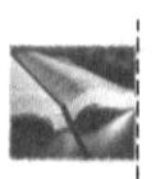 *people shall be separated from thy bowels; and one people shall be stronger than the other people; and the elder shall serve the younger.* **Genesis 25:23**

The two nations referred to in the above Scripture are the Israelites (Jacob's descendants) and the Edomites (Esau's descendants). Hostility and conflict subsequently characterized the relationship between these two nations.

It was customary that the younger of the two sons would serve the older. In this case, however, God reversed the pattern.

This illustrates the principle that a person's place in God's redemptive plan and purpose is not determined by his or her heritage or good works.

God freely chooses to save whomever He wills. This choice of God is an act of grace. God's overflowing compassion cannot be earned or controlled by human beings. He has willed to have mercy upon all.

Take Time Out to Pray

1. Father I thank You for entrusting my womb with great children. I thank You because my womb is the warehouse of great destinies, in the Name of Jesus.

2. O God, I thank you for the products of my womb and I declare that they are fearfully and wonderfully made in Jesus' Name.

3. I receive grace and ease to bring forth children that are admirable, loving and great. I receive the grace to bear and rear children with life-changing abilities.

4. According to Jeremiah 29:11, I receive the expected end for my life as a woman and for the children of my womb in the Name of Jesus.

5. Father I boldly declare that my womb is empowered by You to nurture and incubate a godly seed(s). Therefore, everything that

proceeds from my womb is godly.

6. By Your mercy O God, deliver me and my seed from any harvest of the seed of iniquity sown in the past, in the Name of Jesus.

7. Father I pray today that my case shall stand out for dumbfounding success in Jesus' Name. Amen.

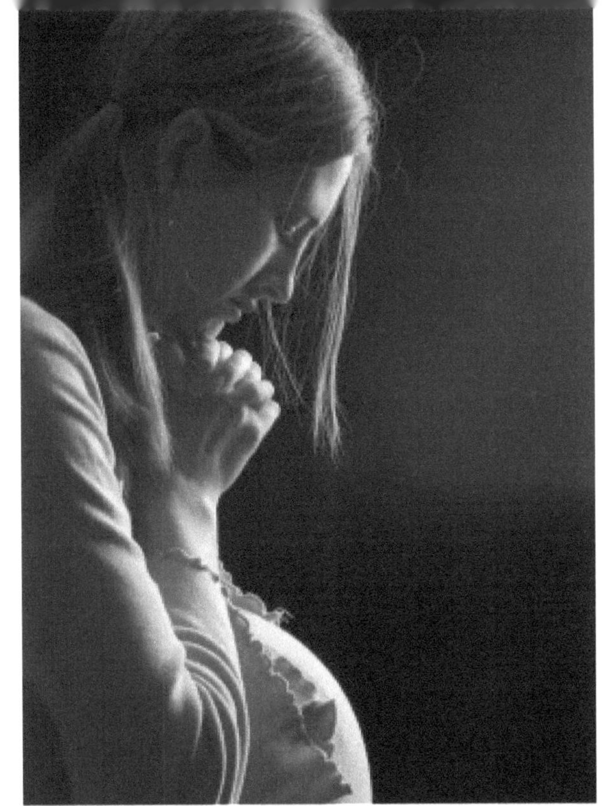

Chapter 2

THE POWER OF
THE WOMB

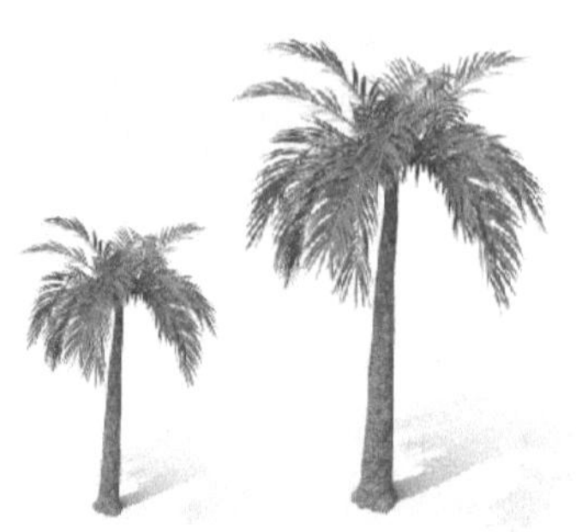

And the LORD said unto her, Two nations are in thy womb, and two manner of people shall be separated from thy bowels; and the one people shall be stronger than the other people; and the elder shall serve the younger.

Genesis 25:23

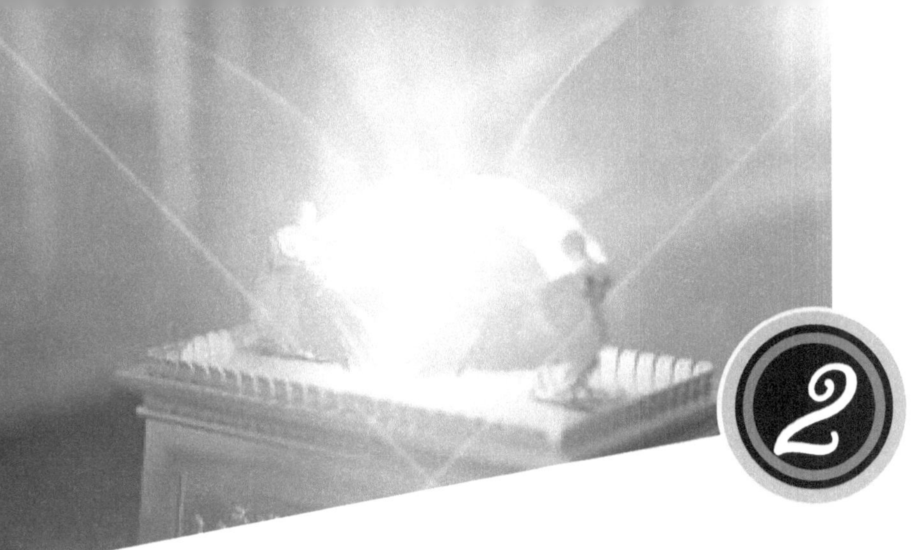

THE POWER OF THE WOMB

" The womb is the centre of every woman's power and creativity. It is where women hold their stories and give birth to their visions. "

It seems that most men and women are "in the dark" about this beautiful mystery within each woman - the womb. Beginning with the anatomy and physiology of the womb, we realize that the uterus (womb) is the strongest muscle in the body, equal in strength only to the heart.

In some native tribal cultures, like the Edo's, Yoruba's etc. women were known as the ones with two hearts, because the womb is seen as a second heart.

The uterus is held in place by many ligaments that extend outward toward the front, sides, and back of a woman's body. It should, however, be understood that the womb is not merely the muscle of the uterus, it is the sacred space within the belly of a woman.

The womb is the centre of each woman's power and creativity. It is where women hold their stories and give birth to their visions.

The womb must be well protected and cared for in order for a woman to achieve the full expression of her creative power.

All through Scripture, God demonstrates the creative power of the womb by the products of the womb of women who knew Him:

1

THE WOMB OF SARAH AT THE AGE OF NINETY INCUBATED AND BROUGHT FORTH A CHILD OF PROMISE.

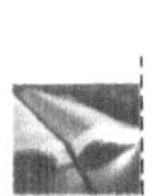

And the LORD visited Sarah as he had said, and the LORD did unto Sarah as he had spoken. For Sarah conceived, and bare Abraham a son in his old age, at the set time of which God had spoken to him.
Genesis 21:1-2

2

THE BIBLE TELLS US THAT REBECCA CARRIED TWO NATIONS IN HER WOMB.

And the LORD said unto her, Two nations are in thy womb, and two manner of people shall be separated from thy bowels; and the one people shall be stronger than the other people; and the elder shall serve the younger.
Genesis 25:23

3

SAMSON'S MOTHER WAS VISITED BY AN ANGEL WHO TOLD HER THAT HER WOMB WILL CARRY A MOST-NEEDED DELIVERER IN ISRAEL.

And there was a certain man of Zorah, of the family of the Danites, whose name was Manoah; and his wife was barren, and bare not. And the angel of the LORD appeared unto the woman, and said unto her, Behold now, thou art barren, and bearest not: but thou shalt conceive, and bear a son. Now therefore beware, I pray thee, and drink not wine nor strong drink, and eat not any unclean thing: For, lo, thou shalt conceive, and bear a son; and no razor shall come on his head: for the child shall be a Nazarite unto God from the womb: and he shall begin to deliver Israel out of the hand of the Philistines.

Judges 13:2-5

THE **LORD** ANNOUNCED THAT **ELIZABETH** WOULD CARRY A SPECIAL BABY IN HER WOMB.

This special baby would be the forerunner of the Saviour of the world.

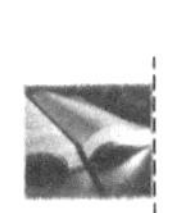

But the angel said unto him, Fear not, Zacharias: for thy prayer is heard; and thy wife Elisabeth shall bear thee a son, and thou shalt call his name John.

Luke 1:13

THE **LORD** TOOK PERMISSION FROM A YOUNG VIRGIN CALLED **MARY**.

He manifested His brilliance when He used her womb to give birth to the Saviour of humanity.

And the angel came in unto her, and said, Hail, thou that art highly favoured, the

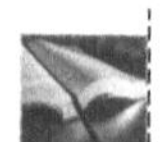 *Lord is with thee: blessed art thou among women. And when she saw him, she was troubled at his saying, and cast in her mind what manner of salutation this should be. And the angel said unto her, Fear not, Mary: for thou hast found favour with God. And, behold, thou shalt conceive in thy womb, and bring forth a son, and shalt call his name JESUS. He shall be great, and shall be called the Son of the Highest: and the Lord God shall give unto him the throne of his father David: And he shall reign over the house of Jacob for ever; and of his kingdom there shall be no end.* **Luke 1:28–33**

By Mary submitting to the will of God, she became the dwelling place for God. Mary's womb was a perfect, rich, fertile, and fruitful soil, totally receptive to, and available for the seed. In Luke 1:42 Elizabeth said, *"Blessed is the fruit of your womb Jesus."*

All the women cited in this chapter were women who placed value on their womb.

The power of the womb can be harnessed by God or satan depending on how each woman handles herself and her relationship with God.

Sarah, Rebecca, Manoah's wife, Elizabeth and Mary, all had something in common – they heard from God. In essence, the creative power of a woman's womb has a whole lot to do with the Creator Himself. A relationship with God boosts the creative power of the womb.

Christian women who know the value and power of their womb can always lay their hands on their womb when praying for their children. This can go a long way to bless and grace the future of their children. This is a good case of the spiritual power inherent in a woman's womb.

Take Time Out to Pray

1. Father I receive unto myself, as a woman, strength, power, might and the anointing of the Holy Spirit, in the Name of Jesus.

2. Heavenly Father, as the womb of Sarah at the age of ninety incubated and brought forth a child of promise, I pray that the children of my womb shall fulfill Your promises. Let Your visitation in my life be made visible in the Name of Jesus.

3. O Lord, Sarah's womb was dead but You revived it. Father, let the Blood of Jesus quicken all that is dead within me. Let all sucked, sapped and paralyzed spiritual milk and strength of my life resurrect by the Blood of Jesus, in Jesus' Name.

4. O God, as Rebecca carried two nations in her womb, I declare that I am a mother of nations – nations that shall birth the glory of my God in their generation.

6. Heavenly Father, I bind the spirit of error that was manifested in Esau and led to the loss of his birthright. The spirit of error shall never be a part of the life of the children of my womb, in the Name of Jesus.

7. Lord I declare that as Manoah's wife was visited by an angel who told her that her womb will carry a most-needed deliverer, so shall it be with my life. I pray O God that every child that passes through my womb shall fulfill Your Divine agenda on earth, in Jesus' Name.

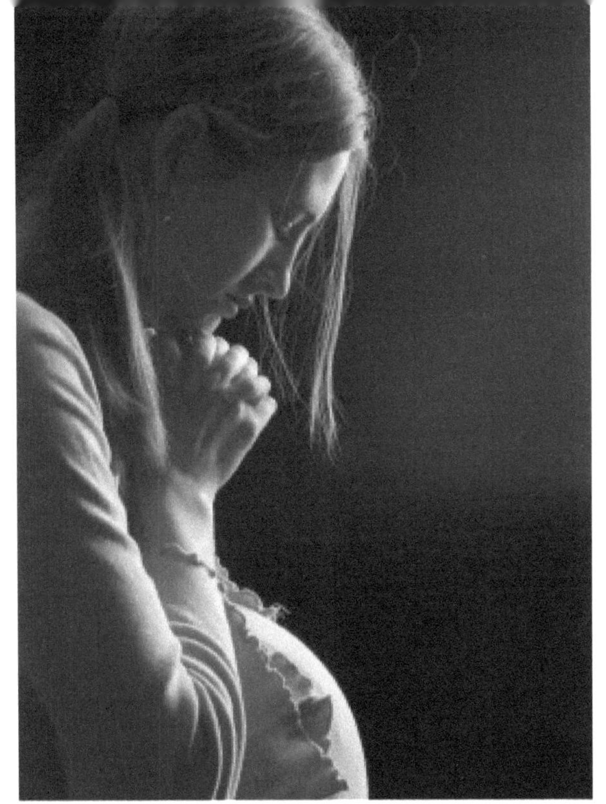

Chapter 3

THE WOMB AS
AN ALTAR

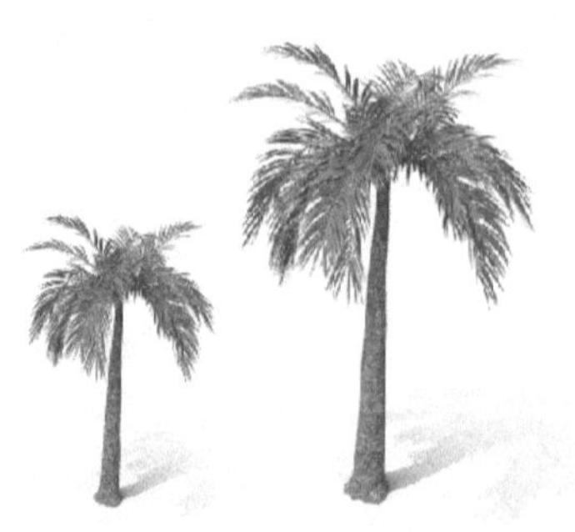

"
For thou hast possessed my reins: thou hast
covered me in my mother's womb.

Psalms 139:13
"

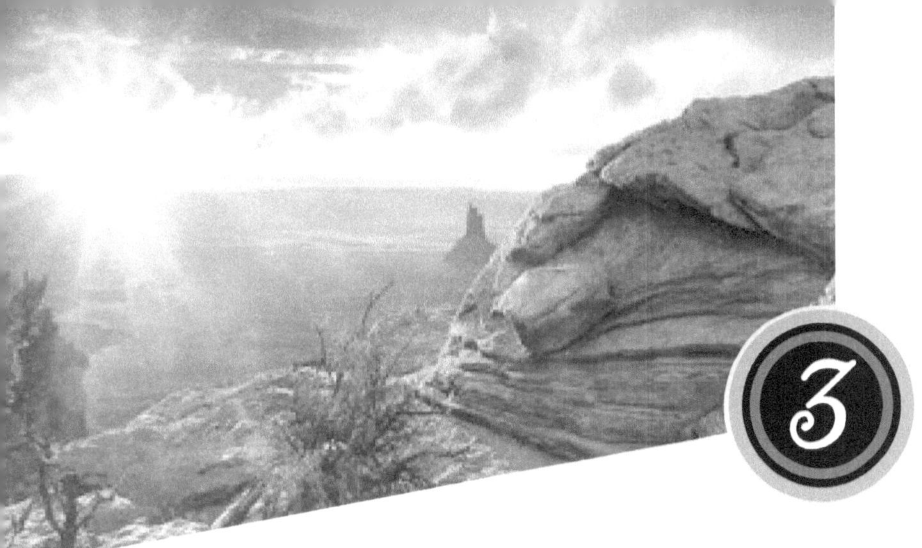

THE WOMB AS AN ALTAR

> **Once the womb altar is desecrated, the product will, of a necessity, be corrupt.**

One very obvious reason why a woman's womb exudes such creative power is because it can also act as an altar.

A major definition of an altar is, "a place of covenant." All the covenants that God made with men were made before specific altars. So, the altar is a place where humanity and Divinity meet; a place where humanity cuts covenants with Divinity.

> **The womb acts as a meeting point between humanity and Divinity.**

In Jeremiah 1:5, God had said to the prophet Jeremiah, *"Before I formed thee in the belly I knew thee; and before thou camest forth out of the womb I sanctified thee, and I ordained thee a prophet unto the nations."*

Here, the womb of Jeremiah's mother acted as the meeting point of covenant between God and her unborn child.

From the story of Prophet Jeremiah, we discover that new life begins with God and He has His eye on the baby in the womb.

Also, the womb of the Apostle Paul's mother acted as a meeting point between God and her unborn child.

Paul attests to the fact that God separated him from his mother's womb and called him by His grace.

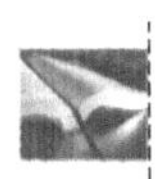

But when it pleased God, who separated me from my mother's womb, and called me by his grace,... **Galatians 1:15**

Again, the Psalmist explains that he had an encounter with God in the womb. He says that God had shaped him in the womb even before bringing him out.

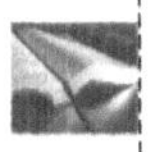

Oh yes, you shaped me first inside, then out; you formed me in my mother's womb.
Psalms 139:13, MSG

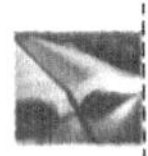

For thou hast possessed my reins: thou hast covered me in my mother's womb.
Psalms 139:13

This is a mystery which will help us to understand why, like every other altar, the womb should be accepted and treated as sacred.

In most churches, the altar is a place specially adorned. Most times, it is a special platform from which the preacher gives sermons. This part of the church is reserved for uncommon use. It is believed to be the holiest part of the church.

The church is a great temple and life exudes from the messages given on the altar. A woman's body is also a temple of the Holy Spirit and the womb is the altar of that temple that brings forth a new life into the world.

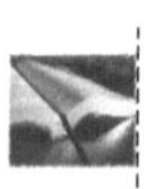

What? know ye not that your body is the temple of the Holy Ghost which is in you, which ye have of God, and ye are not your own? **1Corinthians 6:19**

A woman's womb should be seen as a most sacred part of the woman's body. The Bible talks about the fact that the members of our bodies are actually the members of Christ.

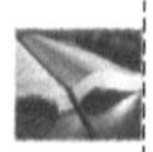

Know ye not that your bodies are the members of Christ? shall I then take the

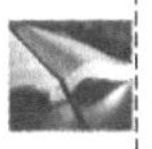 *members of Christ, and make them the members of an harlot? God forbid.*
1Corinthians 6:15

Wherever and whenever women were ignorant of this truth or took it for granted, the result was always unpleasant. Once the altar is polluted, what comes from it will be polluted.

The Apostle Paul had said that the members of Christ cannot be made the members of an harlot.

Once the womb altar is desecrated, the product will, of a necessity be corrupt.

MOAB AND AMMON

In Genesis 19:30–38, for instance, Moab and Ammon were born - two bastard nations, crooked, perverse, and godless. They were products of incest. Deuteronomy 23:2 declares that no bastard can enter into the congregation of the Lord, even to the 10th generation.

Do you not know that children born from defiled wombs are products of sexual immorality, and perpetuate wickedness, and much violence?

The reproach of being a bastard makes them to be brutally cruel and aggressive. They desire to conceal the defects in their family of origin.

JUDAH

The scepter of rulers in Israel was given to Judah in Genesis 49:10, but because of sexual immorality (incest), which he committed in Genesis 38, the destiny of the nation was delayed for ten generations. Israel had no king for a long time.

Sexual immorality is capable of destroying the destiny of a whole nation.

Prostitution and witchcraft go hand-in-hand. Sin never exists in isolation. Those who give themselves over to sexual immorality are opening up their lives to being controlled by demonic spirits.

Please meditate on the Scripture below:

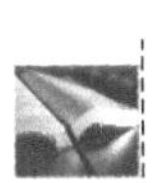

Because of the multitude of the whoredoms of the well favoured harlot, the mistress of witchcrafts, that selleth nations through her whoredoms, and families through her witchcrafts.

Nahum 3:4

JEPHTHAH

In Judges 11:1–3, Jephthah was disinherited, embarrassed and cast out because he was the product of a harlot's womb.

How many of our children have been disinherited because of sexual immorality?

Many!

ABRAHAM AND HAGAR

Do you remember the story of Abraham and Hagar? The Jews, and indeed, the whole world are still battling with the product of that unholy relationship.

SODOM AND GOMORRAH

Do you know also that God destroyed Sodom and Gomorrah because of sexual immorality?

What business are you doing with your womb? Do you not know that your body is the temple of God?

Know ye not that ye are the temple of God, and that the Spirit of God dwelleth in you? If any man defile the temple of God, him shall God destroy; for the temple of God is holy, which temple ye are.
1 Corinthians 3:16–17

And what agreement hath the temple of God with idols? for ye are the temple of the living God; as God hath said, I will dwell in them, and walk in them; and I will be their God, and they shall be my people.
2Corinthians 6:16

Do you not know that abortion is equivalent to murder? The Bible forbids us from shedding innocent blood. Exodus 20:13 says, *"You shall not murder"*.

God superintends over the life in the womb. The life in the womb is precious and so must not be tampered with, at all.

For thou hast possessed my reins: thou hast covered me in my mother's womb. I will praise thee; for I am fearfully and wonderfully made: marvellous are thy works; and that my soul knoweth right well. My substance was not hid from thee, when I was made in secret, and curiously wrought in the lowest parts of the earth.

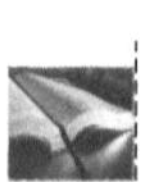 *Thine eyes did see my substance, yet being unperfect; and in thy book all my members were written, which in continuance were fashioned, when as yet there was none of them.* **Psalms 139:13–16**

Every altar is holy unto the Lord, including the womb. When a strange fire is offered on the altar, it attracts the wrath of the consuming fire Himself (Leviticus 10:1).

In like manner, strange fires could be introduced in the womb by the following forms of sexual perversion:

- bestiality;
- lesbianism;
- fornication;
- adultery;
- prostitution; and
- masturbation.

Ungodly seeds are introduced into the womb through illegal sexual relationships.

Some products of polluted wombs include, armed robbers, kidnappers, drug addicts, school dropouts, fraudsters, thugs, militants, ungrateful children, stubborn or disobedient children, aggressive and rude children, etc.

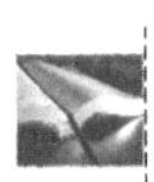

Even from birth the wicked go astray; from the womb they are wayward and speak lies. **Psalms 58:3,** NIV

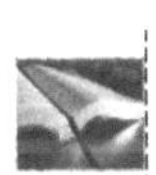

He that committeth sin is of the devil; for the devil sinneth from the beginning. For this purpose the Son of God was manifested, that he might destroy the works of the devil. **1John 3:8**

Every woman must understand that her womb is an altar and thus, should not be defiled in any way.

Just like every other altar, the womb altar is a holy place. No strange fire should be offered on it.

CONSEQUENCES OF SEXUAL IMMORALITY / POLLUTED WOMB

Some men and women indulge in pre-marital sex which is against the Word of God. The Bible clearly states that we should not commit fornication, adultery or any other sexually immoral activity. Disobedience against the Word of God is a sin that destroys a person's destiny. Dreams have been shattered, denied and diverted because of sexual immorality.

Listed herein are consequences of polluting the womb:

A. DEATH

The wages of sin is death. When you indulge in the sin of fornication and adultery, you are sexually dead to yourself. Some people have contracted Sexually Transmitted Diseases (STD) through sex. This has resulted in their untimely death. You not only die physically, you may also die spiritually if you do not repent.

B. FEELING OF GUILT

When you are involved in sexual immorality, you feel guilty. Most times, you commit adultery because you want to satisfy your emotional desire, but in your heart you are filled with guilt for committing fornication and adultery, and that will always hunt you.

C. WASTE OF TIME

Every time you put into premarital sex or sexual immorality is *wasted time*. You waste your time, energy and blood while engaging in sinful acts. You also introduce delay into your marital destiny.

D. DIMINISHED EFFECTIVENESS

Most youths waste their youthful life engaging in pre-marital sex. This diminishes their performance and effectiveness in being active in sex when the right time comes (during marriage). For married men and women, when they indulge in sexual immorality (adultery), it weakens the performances with their spouses.

E. ABORTION

Pre-marital sex leads to unwanted pregnancy. Unwanted pregnancy could end up in abortion. Abortion is a sin of murder.

F. DISOBEDIENCE TO GOD'S WORD

The Word of God says we should not commit fornication or adultery. The Word of God says we should not kill or lie. When you get involved in sexual immorality, you are disobeying God's Word. That disobedience will lead to further sins like carrying out an abortion (murder).

G. FRAGMENTED FUTURE

Most men and women have had their dreams aborted, future fragmented and plans shattered, just because of a few minutes of sexual immorality.

H. DAMAGE TO ONE'S WOMB

Some married women today cannot get pregnant because of the damage done to their womb. Some of them got involved in sexual immorality, which resulted in an unwanted pregnancy. This eventually led to an abortion that damaged the womb.

I. SIN AGAINST YOUR OWN BODY

The Bible says that our body is the temple of the Living God. When you get involved in fornication or adultery, you are sinning against your body, which is the temple of God.

J. BAD MARITAL FOUNDATION

Some married couples cannot count the number of boys or girls with whom they had sexual intercourse before marriage. This trend causes a lot of problems after marriage. They begin to compare their spouse's sexual performances with those of the immoral sex hawkers they mingled with before marriage. This is one reason why some men still engage in extra-marital affairs.

K. BREEDING OF BASTARDS

Some children are products of illicit sexual relationships that were not meant to be.

L. DAMAGE OF REPRODUCTIVE ORGAN

There are a lot of sexually transmitted diseases today. Some men have lost the ability to impregnate their wives because of Sexually Transmitted Diseases which have destroyed their sexual organs.

M. WRONG MARRIAGE

Some women today have ended up marrying the wrong person because they became pregnant before marriage. They were forced by their parents to get married to avoid disgrace and shame to their families.

N. LEADS TO POLYGAMY

Some men are married to more than one wife today because they cannot hold their sexual desires. They are forced to marry more than one wife, because they impregnated another woman.

O. PROSTITUTION

Many young ladies today are into sex hawking because they got involved in sexual immorality.

Take Time Out to Pray

1. O Lord I repent of every wrong way I have treated my womb as a secular rather than a sacred gift from you. I ask for forgiveness today in the Name of Jesus and for cleansing through the Blood of Jesus.

2. I command every ancestral covenant affecting the quality of my life to break its hold in the Name of Jesus Christ.

3. Father I make demands on Your mercy over the consequences of my past life, in the Name of Jesus Christ.

4. Any evil covenants prospering in my family, that will not allow young women to get married in purity and in a legitimate way, break and loose your hold in the Name of Jesus Christ.

5. I rededicate my womb as an altar unto my God, in the Name of Jesus Christ.

6. I receive abundant grace to keep my womb unpolluted and my life unspotted from the world in Jesus' Name. Amen.

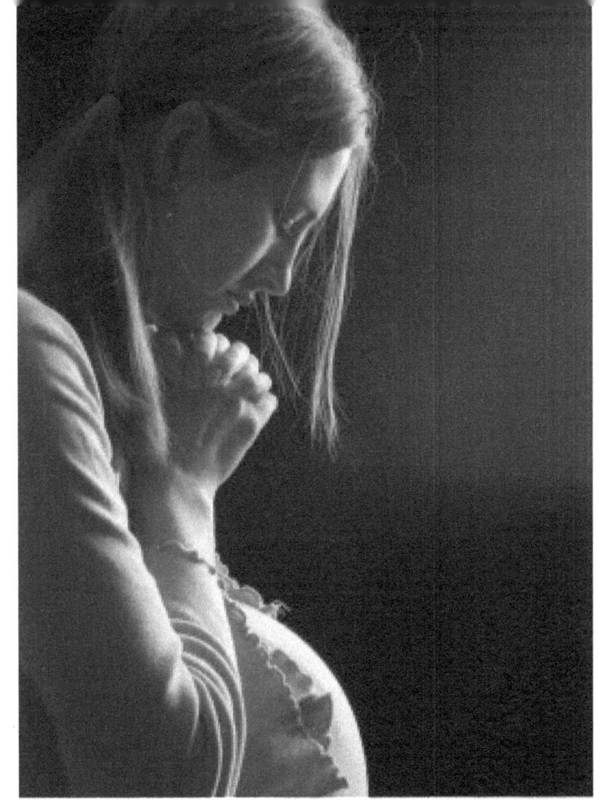

Chapter 4

SHAPING THE UNBORN CHILD

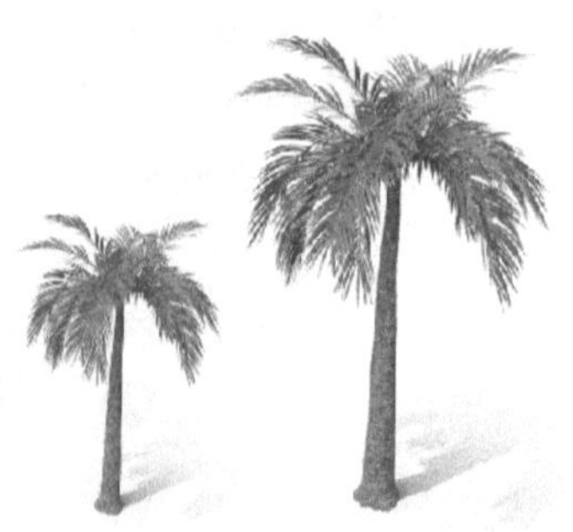

Before I formed thee in the belly I knew thee; and before thou camest forth out of the womb I sanctified thee, and I ordained thee a prophet unto the nations.

Jeremiah 1:5

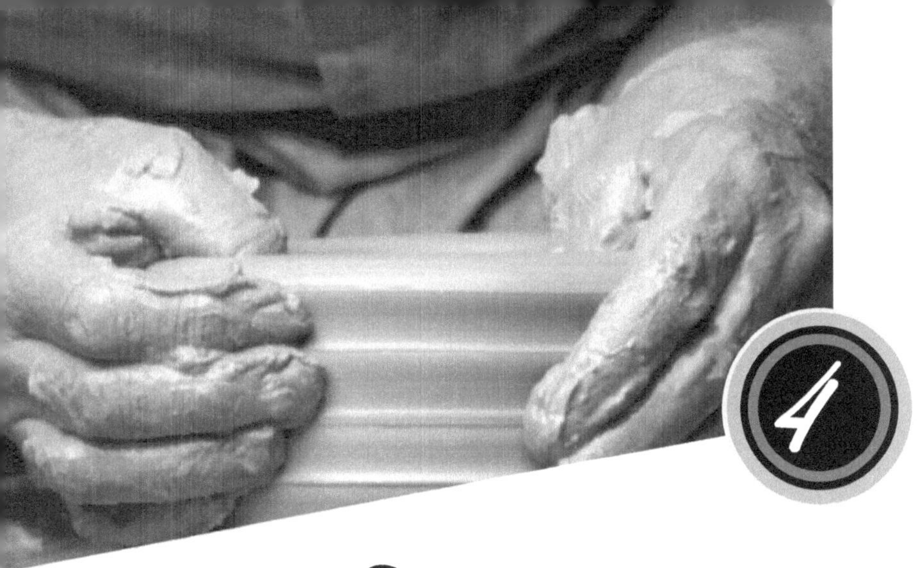

SHAPING THE UNBORN CHILD

> "A child's physical and emotional health is being shaped before it is even born."

The physical and emotional health of a foetus is shaped by the parents' environment and their emotional well-being. That is why it is vital to always confess loving, positive words, especially from the Scriptures, to the foetus throughout the pregnancy. Doing this helps ensure a happy, healthy, and confident child.

A corollary to this discovery is that what a child feels and perceives begins shaping his attitudes and expectations about himself. Whether he ultimately sees himself and hence, acts as a happy or sad, aggressive or meek, secure or anxiety-ridden person depends, in part, on the messages he gets about himself, while he was in the mother's womb.

HOW PARENTS THOUGHTS SHAPE THE LIFE OF THEIR UNBORN CHILD

At a stage during pregnancy, what a mother feels emotionally is transferred directly to her unborn child. Because of this, constant negative emotions can have a damaging effect on the foetus. The foetus absorbs negative emotions like anger, stress or frustration - feelings most adults experience throughout their stressful days.

However, the most harm is done when a mother does not want the child. These and other negative emotions shape the baby's personality.

By the sixth month, the foetus can hear and move in rhythm to its mother's voice.

Imagine the different influence this has if the mother is happily singing or yelling in anger. It is no surprise that sonograms taken while parents yell at each other show the baby's entire body flinching in agitation.

Imagine the damage caused by months of transmitting these negative emotions to a foetus. In fact, studies show that a bad relationship between parents increases the child's risk of psychological and physical damage by a startling 200 percent or more!

Recent studies have shown that six months into a pregnancy, the foetus is already aware, reacting and emotionally active. At six months, the unborn child can see, hear, taste, feel and even learn. So a child's physical and emotional health is being shaped before it is even born. And part of that shaping is determined by how the parents (especially the mother) feel about life and each other.

The following examples shared by a servant of God show how the mother's attitude to her baby in the womb had a detrimental effect upon the baby:

A mother had a terrible experience during the delivery of her second child. This put so much fear into her that when she was pregnant with her third child, she was paranoid about giving birth again and was full of fears. Somehow, these fears entered into the child in the womb. This baby, who is now grown, is still struggling with fears. These fears have plagued her all her life."

A story was told of a backslidden girl who became pregnant. She wanted this child to grow up with a mother and a father and so decided that she would give this baby to a loving family. She was naturally a very loving person, but in order not to get too attached to her baby as she planned to give it away, she thought of it "as nothing" or as a "stone."

However, at the very end of her pregnancy, she met the father of the child again and at the last minute they decided to get married. And so of course, they kept the baby! The baby was born and received with love and joy and was well nurtured by the mother. However, as this baby grew into her second year, she became abnormally affected and screamed with terror if her mother even went out of the room.

Their pastors (the husband had come to the Lord and the wife had been restored to the Lord), prayed about the child's condition. They wondered if she was suffering from rejection of not being accepted during her time in the womb. They prayed over this little child and asked God to heal her from this rejection, and from that moment she never had the problem again.

There is another interesting story mentioned in *The Secret Life of the Unborn Child* by Dr. Thomas Verny:

When this particular baby was born, it would not move its head toward the breast but would turn away. The doctor thought she may be ill, but when she drank milk from the bottle in the nursery, he ruled that out. Next day the same thing happened, so the doctor thought he would try an experiment.

The next day, he gave the sleepy baby to another mother who had consented to try to feed her. Immediately the baby went for the breast and sucked it. The doctor was now more than interested. He went back to the biological mother and asked, "Did you want this baby?"

"No," she replied. "I wanted an abortion but my husband wanted the child. That's why I had her."

That was news to the doctor, but not to the baby! She had been rejected and was now rejecting her mother. This is simple – mothering starts in the womb, not just when the baby is born.

DADDY'S FEELINGS

Recent research is also beginning to focus much more on the father's feelings. Until recently, his emotions were disregarded. Latest studies indicate that this view is dangerously wrong. They show that how a man feels about his wife and unborn child is one of the single most important factors in determining the success of a pregnancy.

Throughout the pregnancy, the foetus is affected by the father's feelings toward the mother and their child. That is because the foetus can feel what its parents feel.

> **A woman is her baby's conduit to the world. Everything that affects her, affects the baby.**

When a man abuses or neglects his pregnant wife, it also affects the physical and emotional well-being of the unborn child.

An equally vital factor in the child's emotional well-being is his father's commitment to the marriage.

> **A child hears his father's voice in the uterus, and there is solid evidence that hearing that voice makes a big emotional difference.**

In cases where a man talked to his child in the uterus using short soothing words, the newborn was able to pick out his father's voice in a room, even in the first hour or two of life. More than pick out, the child responds to the father's voice emotionally. If the child is crying, for instance, at the sound of the father's voice he will stop. That familiar, soothing sound from the father gives him the assurance of safety.

As we have seen, soon after conception, a level of consciousness exists in the embryo. A good father-mother relationship is therefore good for the unborn child. This helps create how the child will see itself in its life ahead. For example, it will feel happy or sad, be aggressive or meek, secure or insecure. In simple summary, as a foetus develops, its subconscious stores information to prepare it for its mother's environment.

The father's role in relation to the mother is very important too. With this knowledge at their disposal, mothers and fathers have an unparalleled opportunity to help shape the personality of their unborn child. They can actively contribute to the child's happiness and well-being, not just in uterus, nor in the years immediately following birth, but for the rest of his life.

Another powerful way parents affect their foetus is through their beliefs. Our life is a reflection of our beliefs. These beliefs come from a lifetime of experiences and interactions with other people. Most of these beliefs are subconscious. And they quietly "program" our minds to react to our world. If these beliefs are negative, it programs our minds to be self- defeating.

During the pregnancy, parents who dwell on negative thoughts send these feelings to the foetus. In turn, this instills fear into the child before it even enters the world.

So, whether the mother's thoughts and emotions are positive and reinforcing or negative and rejecting, they are helping to define and shape the child's character. In fact, it is said that at one time or another, nearly every expectant mother senses that she and her unborn child are reacting to one another's feelings.

BONDING WITH THE UNBORN CHILD

From the foregoing, we can establish some simple facts: a womb is where a child stays; a place that offers protection and shelter.

First, the sperm of a man meets with the egg of a woman. After some days, the fertilized ovum goes to settle in the womb and begins to develop little by little.

The processes of mitosis and meiosis take place. That is biology. Then eventually, the head, the legs, the hands, the brain, etc. develop. Everything is formed, but the child remains in the womb to mature until after nine months. Thereafter, a child is brought forth.

A child cannot grow outside the womb. If you are a woman and you do not have a womb, then you may have done something terrible when you were a young girl; and your womb may have been removed as a result. It takes a miracle for you to have another womb. I said 'miracle' because there is nothing that God cannot do. Luke 1:37 tells us that nothing is impossible with God.

What makes me different from a man is that I have something that a man does not have. They are not capable of having it, because they were not created to have it.

But I, Augusta Ogbene, am created with a perfect womb to carry babies. However, I need a man to become pregnant. As powerful as I may suppose I am, I cannot impregnate myself.

I need my husband to give me something that will meet one egg inside of me, to be able to carry a baby. And if the thing that my husband gives me does not enter inside of my womb, the baby will not be formed. There are men and women inside of the man.

The man determines whether I should give birth to girls or boys. I cannot determine it myself.

Those women who are being punished by their husbands because they are giving birth only to female children, should know that it is what the man gives them that they release.

Those men are living in ignorance. The man determines the sex of the baby that the woman brings forth. The woman is merely a receptacle, a receiver. What the man puts inside of her is what she brings forth.

A woman carries something that is sacred. She carries something with a Divine destiny in her womb. This is why I am saying that the womb is like an altar where humanity and Divinity meet.

In the Book of Genesis, the Bible says Rebecca was pregnant, and there was so much commotion in her womb. She looked at herself and said, *"I know I didn't get pregnant in time; but is this how pregnancy worries people? I have been seeing pregnant women; their own is not like this. My own is different. Why is my case like this?"* (Paraphrased)

She had to go for enquiries. It was as if she went to enquire from a woman or man of God. Do not ask me who. But the Bible says she went to make enquiries. And when she got there, she got the message – "Woman, your case is different, because you are carrying two nations." Every man is a nation.

God said, "You are carrying two nations and they are already fighting. They are struggling over who will come out first. They are not ordinary children."

Rebecca's womb was an altar. The children were incubated there and built up. Gradually they grew until the ninth month, when they were given birth to. So is every woman's womb.

A woman's womb is specially designed to carry and bring forth nations - great men and women of destiny.

The story was told of a young mother who got seriously bonded with her unborn baby and today she has a great testimony. When she was pregnant, she came to Nigeria from the UK.

The story has it that in the night or early in the morning, she would get her Bible, sit down and keep it on her laps. She would say, "Baby, it is time for Bible study. Today, we are going to study the Book of…" She would mention the Book, and then she would read it out. She would read out the passage to the baby.

Then, if the baby disturbed, she would say, "You are inconveniencing mummy. Sit down well. So, the baby would sit well. Then she would say, "Listen, be attentive. Listen, this is the Word of God." She would read it. After reading it, she would tell the baby: "So David killed Goliath in the Name of the Lord. Now we use the Name of Jesus. Baby, as you come out, you are going to challenge every Goliath in the Name of Jesus."

This is quite amazing!

This young mother believed that the baby was a spirit and therefore could hear. She said she wanted her baby to get used to the Word of God, so that he would not reject it when he is born.

Then, when she wanted to sleep in the night, she would say, "Baby, it is time to sleep. Let us pray." She would kneel down; then she would keep quiet for a moment. According to her, the quiet moments were the period that 'Baby was praying.' She imagined that the baby was praying his own prayer before she rounded it off herself. This way, she created an endless bond with her baby.

She kept speaking to her baby even after birth. She never considered that her baby was too little to hear because she believed the baby was a spirit. In the morning, she would read the Bible to the baby, before everyone would come together to pray. The baby had his own special Bible.

Today, that baby is over twelve years old, and he is the preacher in their Children Church in the UK. He ministers in the anointing of the Holy Spirit and it baffles everyone. But it all began in the womb.

The womb is really the birthplace of destinies. Psalm 139:16 (TLB) says, "*You saw me before I was born and scheduled each day of my life before I began to breathe. Every day was recorded in your Book!*"

Every godly womb gives birth to a blessed

child. A certain woman appreciating Jesus said in Luke 11:27b, *"Blessed is the womb that bare thee, and the paps which thou has sucked."*

Sometimes, God shuts the womb of a particular woman for a season. This is to get her prepared spiritually, emotionally etc., to carry a child of destiny.

God's destiny for a child begins to manifest right from the womb of a woman.

Some examples are:

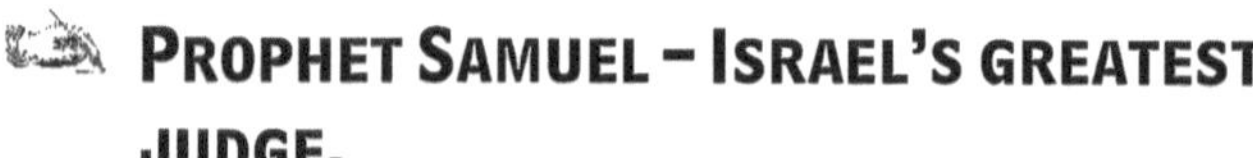

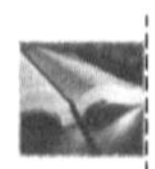 PROPHET SAMUEL – ISRAEL'S GREATEST JUDGE.

Samuel was the product of maternal dedication. Even before he was born, his mother - Hannah, already made up her mind to give Samuel fully and freely back to God.

And Samuel grew and the Lord was with him, and did not let none of his word fall to the ground. **1 Samuel 3:19**

Think about John the Baptist. He was *"filled with the Holy Ghost even **from his mother's womb***" (Luke 1:15 and 16:41).

Paul says that God *"separated me **from my mother's womb**...that I might preach Him among the heathen"* (Galatians 1:15, 16).

Samson said, *"I have been a Nazarite unto God **from my mother's womb**"*(Judges 16:7).

The prophet Isaiah said, *"The Lord hath called me from the womb; **from the bowels of my mother** hath He made mention of my name"* (Isaiah 49:1 and 49:5).

God said of Jeremiah, *"Before thou camest forth **out of the womb**, I sanctified thee and I ordained thee a prophet unto the nations"* (Jeremiah 1:5).

Start praying daily over your baby as soon as you know the wonderful news of conception. As we have seen, the baby in uterus is able to hear. This is an important time to speak lovingly to the baby and welcome this little one to your family. It is time to start reading the Word of God to your baby. It is a good time for the baby to get to know the father's voice.

Women must recognize the power of their wombs and use their knowledge positively to shape the life of their unborn children.

FIVE REASONS WHY THE UNBORN CHILD NEEDS PRAYER

Praying for the baby while still in the womb has long term benefits: Some of which are:

1. *It sets in motion a path to guide the child through life.*

2. *It provides an opportunity to pray out of the child's life unpleasant patterns flowing through the family line such as immorality, drunkenness, lying, disobedience, stealing, poverty, etc.*

3. It offers the chance to present the child to God as a living sacrifice.

4. It is time to secure the child in Christ and pray the prayer of salvation on its behalf.

5. It presents an avenue where the life, destiny, attitude, character and future of the child can be moulded into Biblical shape.

It is recommended to say prayers from conception to delivery of the child. The prayers can be said in the morning, afternoon and evening.

Take Time Out to Pray

1. By Your mercy, O God, deliver me and the child(ren) of my womb from any harvest of the seeds of iniquity sown in the past or present, in the Name of Jesus.

2. Father, by faith in Your Word, I cut off every unpleasant pattern flowing through my family line, such as immorality, drunkenness, lying, disobedience, stealing, poverty etc.

3. Lord I dedicate and present the children of my womb to You as living sacrifices.

4. I pray today that my children shall yearn for the salvation of God through Christ Jesus.

5. I declare that the destiny of my children shall be moulded by the Holy Spirit in Jesus' Name. Amen!

6. Abba Father, help my children to love and serve You always in Jesus' Name.

7. Let the Spirit of excellence and distinction rest upon my children. Lord direct them in all their undertakings in Jesus' Name. Amen.

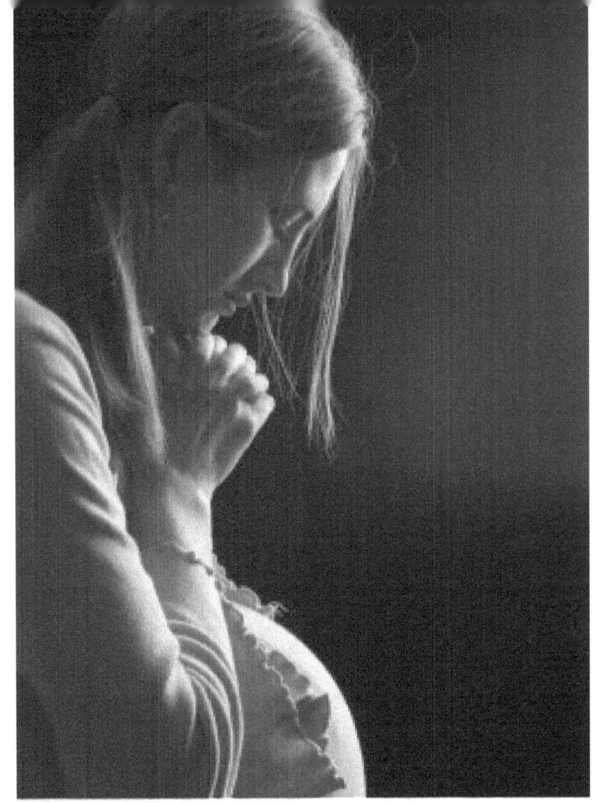

Chapter 5

MANDATE OF
THE WOMB

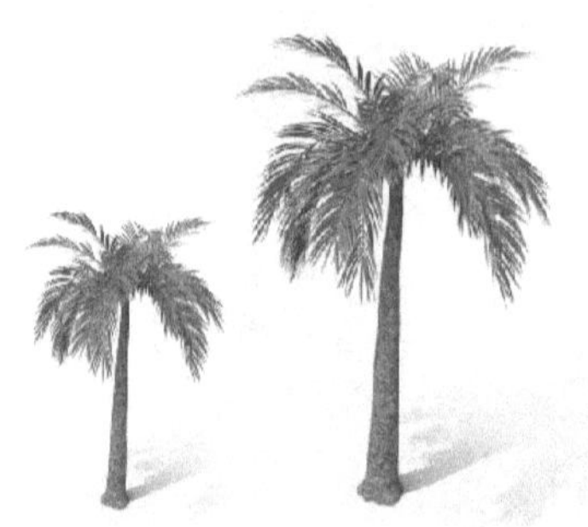

That our sons may be as plants grown up in their youth; that our daughters may be as corner stones, polished after the similitude of a palace:

Psalms 144:12

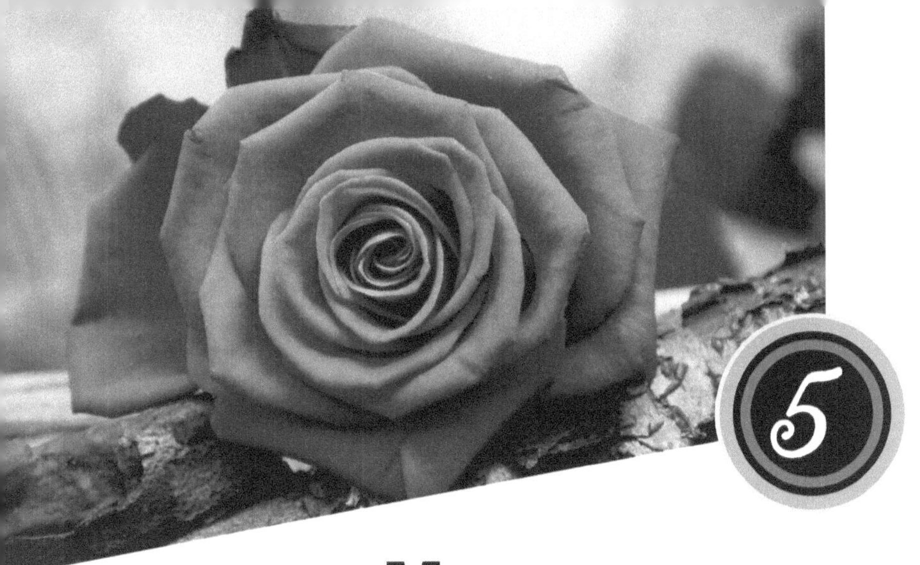

5

MANDATE OF
THE WOMB

> *Home becomes a palace when the
> daughters are maids of honour and the
> sons are nobles in spirit.*

All of God's creation has a particular mandate. There is nothing existing that was not created with a purpose.

When God created the sun and the moon, even as close as their functions seemed, God

97

mandated the sun to give its light in the day and the moon in the night. In the same vein, every creation of man has a specific mandate.

No government office or ministry is created without a specific mandate. In like manner, no one creates or brings forth anything without an underlying purpose.

God created the womb with a specific mandate. One of the mandates of the womb is found in Psalm 144:12, and that is, **TO PRODUCE WHOLESOME CHILDREN.** It says, *"May our sons flourish in their youth like well-nortured plants. May our daughters be like graceful pillars, carved to beautify a palace."*

Wholesome children are children fashioned after all manner of excellence in every sphere of human endeavour. The Bible talks about such children in the Book of Daniel 1:4:

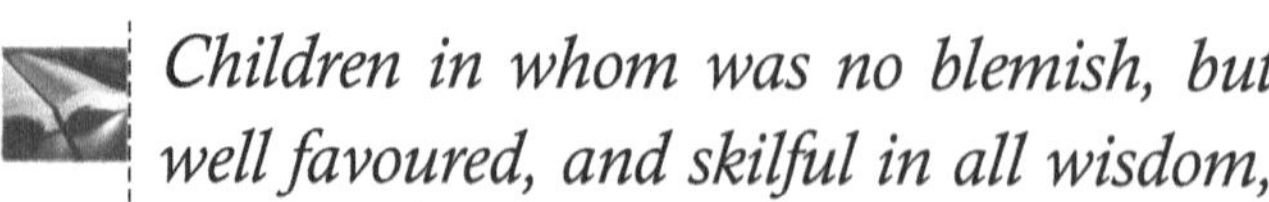

Children in whom was no blemish, but well favoured, and skilful in all wisdom,

and cunning in knowledge, and understanding science, and such as had ability in them to stand in the king's palace, and whom they might teach the learning and the tongue of the Chaldeans.

When King Nebuchadnezzar wanted children who could represent certain principles and practices in his kingdom, he asked that they select from the children of Judah, children who had no blemish, but well favoured, skillful in all wisdom, cunning knowledge, understood science, and had the ability to stand before him.

These were wholesome children. This kind of children could only be gifts from God. They were handsome and beautiful. But that was not all about it. They were not outcasts in society. They were well-favoured and loved. They were not only wise but skillfully wise. In other words, they could apply themselves to so many natural abilities and handle events. They were equally cunning in knowledge, meaning that they were extremely versatile. Much more than these, they were not timid. They were bold children who could stand in the presence of the king.

It is therefore, the mandate of the womb to produce such healthy, wholesome and handsome sons, like strong vigorous plants; and to produce daughters that will be strikingly tall, well proportioned and beautiful, like the sculptured pillars of a palace.

God wants a woman's womb to produce young men that are well-nortured and strong, with great destinies.

Daughters unite families as corner stones join walls together, and at the same time they adorn them as polished stones garnish the structure into which they are built. Home becomes a palace when the daughters are maids of honour, and the sons are nobles in spirit; then the father is a king, and the mother a queen. This makes the home a royal residence/palace.

A city built up of such dwellings is a city of palaces, and a state composed of such cities is a Republic of Princes. We need to examine the products of our womb as mothers to find out if they are fulfilling this original mandate.

One of the greatest joys of a woman is the day she leaves her parents' home and becomes a wife. Next to that is the joy of being a mother. Every normal man or woman has great expectation of becoming a parent someday.

The birth of a child into any home is considered to be a seal of blessing upon that family. Children are the crown of their parents.

If, as a woman, you do not have the fruit of the womb, you have to look at what God has said concerning the fruit of the womb and go to God in prayer. Go to Him and say, "God, You did not create me not to carry babies; you created my womb to carry babies. If my mother gave birth to me, then I must give birth to children." Continuously declare the Word of God over your life:

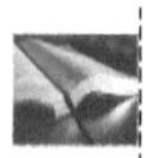 *There shall nothing cast their young, nor be barren, in thy land: the number of thy days I will fulfil.* **Exodus 23:26**

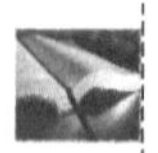 *Thy wife shall be as a fruitful vine by the sides of thine house: thy children like olive plants round about thy table.* **Psalms 128:3**

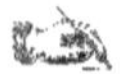 BRINGING FORTH GOD'S REWARD

It is also the mandate of the womb to bring forth God's reward.

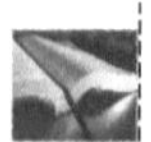 *Children are an heritage of the Lord and the fruit of the womb is His reward.*

Psalms 127:3

Children are an heritage of the Lord. This points to another mandate of the womb, that of building up a house, by leaving descendants to keep our name and family alive upon the earth.

Without this, what is a man's purpose in accumulating wealth? To what purpose does he build a house if he has none in his household to hold the house after him? Yet in this matter a man is powerless without the Lord.

The great Napoleon was childless and so could not create a dynasty. Hundreds of wealthy persons would give half their estates if they could hear the cry of a babe born of their own bodies.

Children are a heritage which Jehovah Himself must give, or a man will die childless, and thus his house will be unbuilt.

God chooses the fruitful womb to reward His

people. So, the fruit of the womb is a reward from God.

God gives children, not as a penalty nor burden, but as a favour. Even with all the limited incomes, our best possessions are our own dear offspring, for whom we bless God every day. It is one of the greatest outward blessings to have a family full of dutiful children.

To have many children is the next blessing to much grace. To have many children about us is better than to have much wealth about us.

To have a store of these olive plants (as the Psalmist calls them) round about our table is better than to have a store of oil and wine upon our table.

We know the worth of dead, or rather lifeless treasures, but who knows the worth of living treasures? Are not houses and lands, gold and silver, a heritage bestowed by the Lord upon

His people? Doubtless they are, for the earth is His, and the fullness of it, and He gives it to the children of men. Though all things are of God, yet all things are not alike of Him: children are more of God than houses and lands.

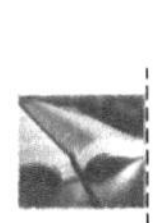

*Ephraim is smitten, their root is dried up, they shall bear no fruit: yea, though they bring forth, yet will I slay even **the beloved fruit of their womb**.* **Hosea 9:16**

God calls children the "dearly beloved fruit of the womb." The context of this passage is that God was going to destroy the "rewards" that He had given them because of their continual disobedience. It shows how God views children and also how the early Hebrews felt about their children.

Ruth 2:12 says, "*The Lord recompense thy work and a full reward be given thee of the Lord God of Israel.*" What was the full reward? Ruth 4:13 gives us the answer: "*The Lord gave her conception and she bare a son.*"

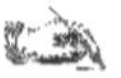 THE WOMB IS A WORKSHOP OF GOD'S CREATION

Isaiah 44:2,24 and 49:5 says, "The Lord that made thee, that formed thee from the womb..." The word *formed* means to be "molded into a form as a potter does." God molds each individual child in the womb. This is a mandate for the womb.

Each woman should yield her womb for God to mold lives. Psalms 139:13-17 (TLB) says, "*You made all the delicate, inner parts of my body, and knit them together* **in my mother's womb.** *Thank you for making me so wonderfully complete! It is amazing to think about. Your workmanship is marvelous.*"

THE WOMB IS A WEAPON AGAINST SATAN

It is the womb that conceives and nourishes the "godly seed" who will come forth to be the light in the darkness and who will destroy the works of Satan in this world.

God is looking for an army. The greatest threat to Satan in this world is godly parents who understand God's intentions and who will bring forth and train a godly seed to fulfill His eternal plans.

The womb is a powerful weapon against Satan. Some women fear to bring babies into this evil world, but this is one of the greatest reasons for having children – to be the light in this dark world!

Therefore, to bear children who will be light in a dark world is a clear-cut mandate of the womb.

And she shall bring forth a son, and thou shalt call his name JESUS: for he shall save his people from their sins. **Matthew 1:21**

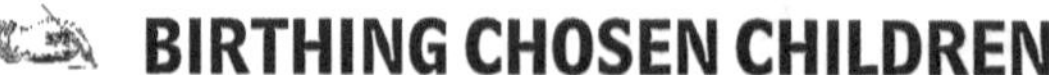

BIRTHING CHOSEN CHILDREN

Ephesians 1:4 tells us that God *"hath chosen us in him before the foundation of the world, that we should be holy and without blame before him in love:"* The destiny of each individual, by Scripture should be that of being holy and blameless before Him in a corrupt world as ours. God expects us to bring forth such children. It is a mandate for the womb of the woman.

God is not expecting the womb to bring forth corrupt and immoral children who will add to the existing curse in the land.

God expects women to bring forth children who will bring salvation to their generation in many spheres of human endeavour.

This is a mandate and must be fulfilled by every womb. Is your womb fulfilling this mandate?

It is one of the greatest blessings, they say, to have godly parents, and also to have godly children.

In spite of the nudity that we see around these days, where our daughters open their stomach, buttocks and breasts, so many of them have remained unmarried.

No decent man wants to marry a naked girl.

To the many of them I see around, I say to them, "You do not need to open anything, because even your face shows that you are beautiful."

I say to the girls, that no responsible man will like to marry a girl that is walking about the streets naked. If I were a man who wants to marry, when I see that you have shown your body to all men, I will not marry you.

Why?

Because you have already become public

property. You have brought out your breasts for everybody to see. That which is supposed to be for your husband and your children, is now public property."

The mandate of the womb is what we have seen in the preceding Scriptures already examined. If you are not fulfilling that mandate, you need to go to God in the place of prayer.

We need to examine the products of our womb as mothers, to find out if they are fulfilling the original mandate.

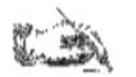

PROTECT YOUR WOMB

Every woman has the responsibility to protect her womb from unexpected attacks and pollution.

Satan hates women with a passion, and this hatred started right from the beginning.

When God laid a curse on Satan, He said, "Satan, there is enmity between you and the woman; between your seed and her seed. The seed of the woman will bruise your head, and you will bruise his heel."

Right from that time, Satan became highly incensed against women. That is why, if you go to churches, you find that women are more possessed. They are easily open to witchcraft spirit, marine spirit, and all kinds of spirits.

The reason is that Satan does not want the woman to be free. Satan's desire is to destroy the seed of the woman. He went after Jesus Christ as a child, thinking he would be able to kill Jesus.

Read Revelation chapter twelve and you will see what Satan tried to do. The serpent that was not dealt with in Genesis, appeared as a dreadful dragon in Revelation.

The problem you do not solve now always waits for you tomorrow. Your "Esau" is by the gate waiting for you.

Some people spend their early days having a good time, but as soon as they want to embrace the future, Esau is there waiting: "You thought I have forgotten what you did to me? Payback time has come."

I pray for you according to Psalms 20:1 - "May the Lord answer you when you're in distress. May the Name of the God of Jacob protect you."

Genesis 3:15 says, *"And I will put enmity between thee and the woman, and between thy seed and her seed. It shall bruise thy head and thou shall bruise his heel."* Satan hates the woman and her seed so much that he uses anything available to him to pollute the womb.

As stated earlier, in the twelfth chapter of the

Book of Revelation, you will see that when the woman was pregnant, everything was going on well. But as she was about to give birth, Satan came immediately and stood by, ready to kill the child.

Satan was like, "Okay, she is going to deliver a man-child; maybe this man-child will come and bruise my head again; therefore, I must kill the man-child."

The Bible says, God helped the woman, and when the devil got to know that God had taken the woman and the child to a place of safety He had prepared, he became very angry. He came against the woman, brought flood and caused much trouble. But the Bible says that the earth helped the woman.

Place your hands on the ground now and declare…

Oh earth, oh earth, oh earth! The Bible tells me, you helped the woman, help me, oh earth! These problems are not for me. I say open up now and swallow up the flood. I say earth, you that helped the woman; I come as the seed of the woman. I command you to open now and swallow up this flood that the enemy has brought against me and my family, in the Name of Jesus. I receive peace today. I receive progress today. I receive success today. I receive blessings today.

Oh earth! Oh earth! Vomit my blessings. Vomit my blessings. Vomit my blessings oh earth! As I stand upon you, I will no longer be stagnant. I will never be stranded in life. I will never become a victim of circumstances, in the Name of Jesus.

I make this declaration today, on behalf of my husband and my children - biological and spiritual. I say oh earth! oh earth! You will not swallow my blessings; but you will swallow all my problems, in the Name of Jesus. Amen.

Take Time Out to Pray

1. I declare that my womb fulfils its mandate. I declare that I do not give birth to ordinary children, but to extraordinarily wholesome children fashioned after all manner of excellence in every sphere of human endeavour, in Jesus' Name.

2. Heavenly Father, I declare that the children of my womb are Children in whom is no blemish, but well favoured, and skilful in all wisdom, and cunning in knowledge, and understanding science, and have the ability in them to withstand pressure, in the Name of Jesus.

3. Every gathering against the success of the fruits of my womb, I command you to scatter by fire in the Name of Jesus.

4. This day, I remove my name and the names of my children from every evil family record, in the Name of Jesus.

5. Heavenly Father, let Your heavenly carpenters nail to death every spiritual robber of my children's progress and prosperity, in Jesus' Name.

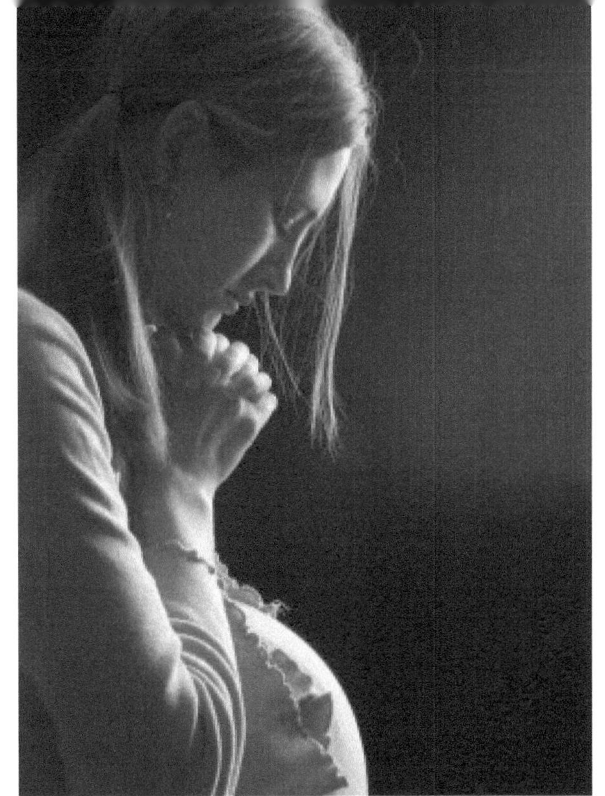

Chapter 6

THE GATEWAY

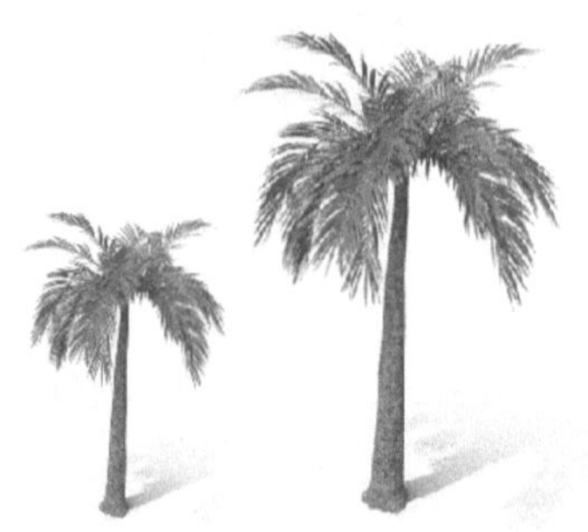

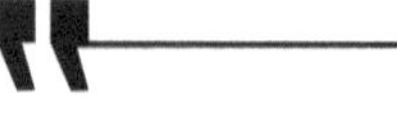

...and brake down the high places of the gates that [were] in the entering in of the gate; keepers of the gates...[were] keepers of the entry.

2Kings 23:2; 1Chronicles 9:19

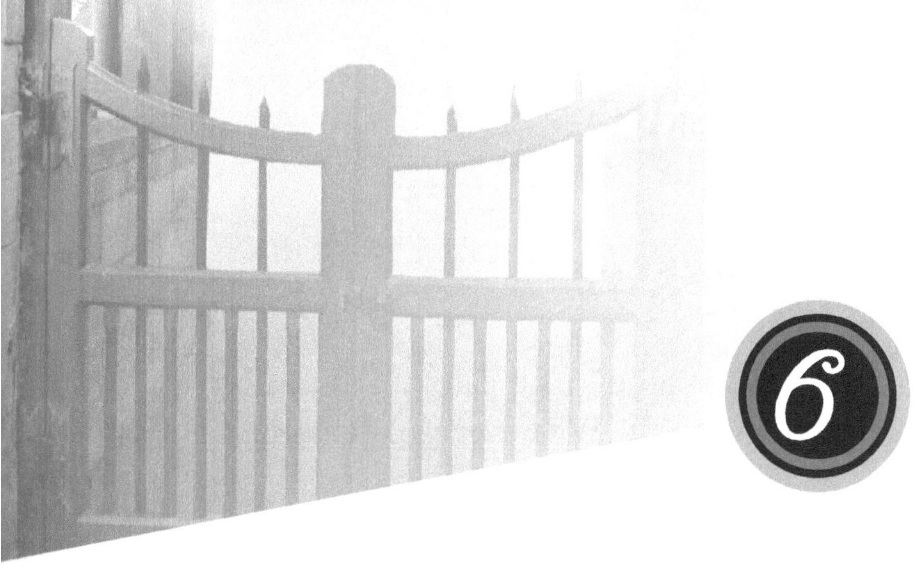

THE GATEWAY

> **Any woman sleeping around with strange men jeopardizes the life and future of her children.**

What is a gateway? It is an access to something. There are several gate ways into the human spirit. Some of these are the eyes, ears, nose, mouth, vagina, and anus. Whatever goes through these human gates determines what will happen to the person's spirit, soul and body.

THE EYE GATE

The eye is a powerful gateway to our body, soul and spirit. Whatever we allow through our eyes will fill our entire being.

> **Until your spiritual eyes are opened, you do not have dominion.**

In Genesis 13:14-17, God said it is what you can see that you can have. Those who are morally depraved keep watching pornography, and their minds are filled with porn images.

Those who watch violent movies have their minds full of violence. Most defiling thoughts are products of what men see. Many sexual perversions are offshoots of what men feed their eyes.

Jesus pointed out that we have the power to choose to look at wholesome and good things. That way, we will be "full of light", shining like a lamp. This, in turn, will help us get our thoughts focused on Godly things instead of sinful things.

Paul wrote, *"Finally, brothers, whatever things is true, whatever is noble, whatever is right, whatever is pure, whatever is lovely, whatever is admirable; if anything is excellent or praise worthy, think about such things"* (Philippians 4:8 NIV).

THE EAR GATE

Just like the eyes, the ears are the gateways into a man's spirit. The Apostle Paul said that faith comes by hearing. That means the amount of faith build up in the life of a man is proportionate to how much of God's Word he hears.

Because the ears are a major gateway to a man's spirit, apart from faith, other emotions can also be stirred by hearing. For instance, fear also comes by hearing.

Seven times in the Book of Revelation, God repeated Himself: "*He who has ears, let him hear what the Spirit is saying to the churches.*" This means that some people may have ears but never hear. The ear gate of their ears may be shut.

The ear gate is very crucial because, according to Romans 10:17, *faith comes by hearing and hearing by the Word of God.* What you hear can determine what you will become. Faith comes by hearing. It is the door to deliverance.

Psalms 107:20 says, "*He sent his word, and healed them, and delivered them from their destructions.*"

How do you receive the Word?

Through the ear-gate.

The ear gate is the door to blessing. It is the door to prosperity.

In Genesis 18:9-14, God spoke, and Sarah heard. She laughed. And from that day on, she kept on laughing. Once you hear what God says, you can be sure it will come to pass.

THE MOUTH GATE

The mouth is also a major gateway into the body. As a matter of fact, most people are defiled by what they take in through their mouth.

Most children have been defiled in the womb because of what their mothers took during pregnancy.

But, can a person really be defiled by what he or she eats?

Can there be spiritual complications because

of what a person takes in?

The answer is, yes.

Medical science tells us that what a pregnant woman eats can affect the life of the baby in the womb through the placenta.

Dr. D. K Olukoya tells the story of a pregnant woman who was a drunkard. Her baby shared some of the alcohol on a regular basis. When the baby was born, it was later detected that the nerves of the baby were already addicted to alcohol and that the baby was crying because its nerves were not getting a regular supply of alcohol which it used to get in the womb.

This is a perfect example of the fact that whatever the mother eats or drinks can affect the child in the womb. And if this is true, we should know that spiritually unclean foods can also affect the spiritual make up of a baby.

In Judges 13:13-14, the angel of the Lord instructing Manoah, said to him, "*Your wife must be careful to do everything I told her to do. She must not eat anything that comes from the grapevines, drink any wine or liquor, or eat any unclean food. She must be careful to do everything I commanded.*"

If Manoah's wife ate anything that came from the grapevines, drank any wine or liquor, or ate any unclean food, it would have adverse effects on the child who was to be born. In other words, it would affect the spiritual make up of the child.

Mothers have to be very careful about what they eat. The mouth is a major gateway to the womb.

Many women, during pregnancy, drink concoctions from juju priests. Some drink *satanic holy water* and *camphor water*. Others even eat demonic food in order to protect their pregnancies, while they inadvertently harm themselves and their unborn child. I have read that many mothers have swallowed eggs given to them by satanic prophets. Others have eaten witchcraft foods and drank blood.

A lot of these things have become evil deposits that have affected their children, some of which are born with very strange manners. Such children found it difficult to change, no matter how much they were corrected.

Another important aspect of the mouth gate is what mothers confess during pregnancy.

It is important to always maintain a positive outlook during pregnancy.

The words of a mother can affect the child in the womb. If the mother is in a praise mood, the child will be, but if the mother is in a negative mood and confesses same, it will also affect the life of the child in the womb.

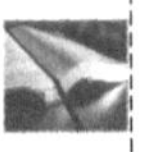 *Bless the LORD, O my soul: and all that is within me, bless his holy name.* **Psalms 103:1**

THE REPRODUCTIVE GATE

The major gateway to a woman's womb is the vagina. Now, for the purpose of avoiding being vulgar, I will use the expression 'private part.'

The private part is one of the major gateways to the womb. Once the private part is defiled with sexual immorality, a woman produces the wrong children - armed robbers, violent and wayward children, militants, cultists, and ungrateful children.

We do many things in ignorance. We always believe nobody is watching, and that it does not matter. "Is it not just for five minutes, and I will come out?" we hear people say. Well, it is true, but there are certain laws that cannot be broken, particularly, the married women that indulge in sexual immorality. Any woman that is sleeping around with strange men is jeopardizing the lives of her children.

We have some traditions in Africa that we must preserve. There is nothing like, "I am born again, old things are passed away; I can commit adultery." That is not true. God's Word does not make any provision for Christians to live in sin. There is eternal damnation awaiting all sinners who refuse to repent.

If you are a woman, not properly married; your husband has not paid dowry on your head, you are in trouble. You simply packed your things to a man's house and said you are in love with each other. And nobody can stop you. Your parents may have warned you, but you disobeyed them. You must formalize that relationship if not it remains illicit.

If you have children from this type of relationship, they are called bastards. Watch out, such children have the tendency to rebel against their parents.

There are certain laws that cannot be ignored. When you ignore or break them, you must prepare your mind to face the consequences.

That man you are living with is not your husband; he is your boyfriend. A man is your boyfriend until he has paid your dowry.

Tell him you do not want to give birth to bastard children.

Tell him you do not want to give birth to armed robbers or militants.

Tell him to go and pay your dowry, so that the blessing of God will come upon your children.

Some people think it is too late because they already have children. No it is not. Go and regularize that relationship.

Some women are living with men who have driven away their original wife. Such women are in trouble. Now get this: if a man drove away a woman because of you, listen, you are really in trouble.

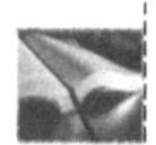 *The women of my people have ye cast out from their pleasant houses;* **from their children have ye taken away my glory forever.** Micah 2:9

Imagine that! The woman that a man has been building his life with, he decides to cast her out. He decides to throw her out.

Please, lift up your hand and pray:

My Father! My Father! Oh my Father! The God of all flesh, it will not be said and it will not be heard, that my husband threw me out from our home. Oh my father! Any demon from his village or from my village that would want to manipulate him, today, I bind that demon, and I cast him into the abyss in the Name of Jesus.

Oh my Father! Your Word says that my husband should not deal with me treacherously. I resist every spirit of treachery in the Name of Jesus. My husband will not betray me. My husband will never reject me. He will never throw my things out. We are joint heirs. We are co-builders. My husband and I believe in the Lord Jesus Christ. And in the long run, we shall be in heaven. No strange woman will take my place in my husband's heart. Every day of my life, my husband will have me in his heart. He will continue to cherish me. He will continue to love me. He will never desire any other woman; in the Name of Jesus.

The second part of that Scripture says, "…from their children, have ye taken away my glory forever." God forbid! Pray now:

My Father! My Father! Oh Father! If there is

anything that happened in my family, that made my children's glory to be taken away, today, I come before you. I buy back my children's glory with the Blood of Jesus; the Blood of Jesus; the Blood of Jesus. Oh my Father, my children resemble you in the Name of Jesus. Amen.

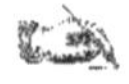 ## SOME ACTS OF SEXUAL PERVERSION IN SOCIETY TODAY

LESBIANISM

This is the act of a woman being attracted to and having sexual relations with another woman. It is a grievous sin against God. Most women appear very beautiful on the outside but are deeply rotten on the inside. Consequently, women sleep with women. They say they do not like men, so a girl will have sexual intercourse with another girl.

They are 'lesbians.' Such people are under the judgment of God.

> *Wherefore, God also gave them up to uncleanness through the lusts of their own hearts, to dishonor their own bodies between themselves; who changed the truth of God into a lie, and served the creature more than the creator, who is blessed forever. Amen. For this cause, God gave them up unto vile affections: For even their women did change the natural use into that which is against nature.*
> **Romans 1:24-26**

If you are a woman, and you love a fellow woman, you have a vile affection. It is an abomination before God.

HOMOSEXUALITY

A homosexual is a person, especially a man, who is sexually attracted to another of the same sex. A homosexual man has sexual relations with another man. In today's world, some men behave like women to attract their fellow men. All these are an abomination before God and have their due punishment.

> *…And likewise also men, leaving the natural use of the woman burned in their lust one towards another; men with men, working that which is unseemly and receiving in themselves that recompense of their error which was meet.* **Romans 1:27**

BESTIALITY

This is sexual activity between a human being and an animal. This is also an abomination before God. I learnt that there are girls who sleep with dogs for a fee. Can you imagine a human being created in God's image and likeness, mating with dogs? This is bestiality and it is an abomination.

Being filled with all unrighteousness,

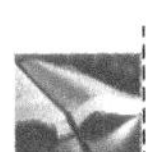

fornication, wickedness,...inventors of evil things,... without natural affection,.. Who knowing the judgment of God, that they which commit such things are worthy of death, not only do the same, but have pleasure in them that do them. **Romans 1:29-32**

The people or churches that encourage such things, have death as their reward. There is a death sentence on anybody that encourages lesbianism, homosexuality, or bestiality. That is the Word of God.

RAPE

This is a sexual assault which can happen to both men and women of any age. It is the penetration, no matter how slight, of the vagina or anus with anybody or object, or oral penetration by a sex organ of another person, without the consent of the victim.

Rape is forced and unwanted. It is about

power, not sex. A rapist uses force or violence or threat to take control over another person. Some rapists use drugs to take away a person's ability to fight back.

Rape is a crime, whether the person committing it is a stranger, an acquaintance or a family member.

Rape is an act of aggression, and violence.

Rape within the family is also a criminal offence, though not often announced. If a thief broke into your home and stole some of your possessions, you would immediately report the crime to the police. But what if someone was able to break into your life and steal your feelings of self-worth, crippled your ability to trust others, beat you hands down until you are bruised with fear?

What if you were a child and that "someone" was your father or brother or uncle or grandfather? No matter how it happened, rape is frightening and traumatizing.

People who have been raped need care, comfort and a way to heal.

2Samuel 13:1-21 describes the rape of Tamar by her half brother Amnon. Tamar was sexually and verbally abused, shamed, and rejected. Tamar was the king's daughter. She was a virgin, she had never engaged in any act of sexual immorality. Out of lust and selfish compulsion based on gratification, Amnon raped her.

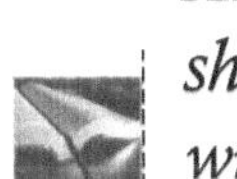

> *Then Amnon hated her with great hatred, the hatred with which he hated her was greater than the love with which he had loved her. And Amnon said to her, "Get up! Go!" but she said to him, "No, my brother, for this wrong in sending me away is greater than the other that you did to me". But he would not listen to her. He called the young man who served him and said, "Put this woman out of my presence and bolt the door after her".*
>
> **2Samuel 13:15-17**

Tamar was thrown out of Amnon's apartment like a piece of dirty rag. She bore the reproach of the rape and lived the rest of her life like a widow.

In Genesis34:1-2, Dinah, the daughter of Jacob and Leah, went to visit some of the women who lived there. She was seen by Hamor's son, Shechem, the leader of the Hivites, and he grabbed her and raped her.

Dinah was an innocent victim. After the rape incident, she was neither comforted nor consulted. Instead, she was treated with almost as much disrespect by her family members as she was by Shechem.

INCEST

This is sexual intercourse between close relatives. It is sexual activities between individuals of close blood relationships, members of the same household, step relatives related by adoption or marriage.

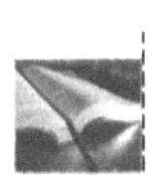 *Cursed be he that lieth with his sister, the daughter of his father, or daughter of his mother.* **Deuteronomy 27:22**

In Genesis 19:30-38, Lot had left Sodom and Gomorrah with his two daughters. Lot was old and his daughters wanted heirs, so they decided to commit incest with their father. This ungodly decision had an adverse impact on the future history of Israel.

Lot's daughters became pregnant by him. They delivered what became two of the greatest adversaries of Israel, the Ammonites and the Moabites. Lot's daughters never took their time to consider the consequences of their incestuous acts. They made a hasty decision and in just two nights, created a seemingly never ending situation for a nation.

According to Deuteronomy 23:4-7, the Israelites were banned from having contacts with these two nations. *"No Ammonite or Moabite or any of their descendants may enter the assembly of the Lord's people, not even in the tenth generation"*.

Take Time Out to Pray

1. Father, let every dirty act or habit standing as an obstacle to God's blessings in my life or the lives of my children, be destroyed totally in the Mighty Name of Jesus Christ.

2. O Lord, I pray today that they shall be ashamed and brought to confusion together that rejoice at my failure or the failure of my seed in life, in the Name of Jesus.

3. O God, any person standing up at midnight to curse me or any member of my family, with the evil habits of pornography, homosexuality, masturbation, lesbianism, etc., I command that they shall be clothed with shame and dishonour in the Name of Jesus.

4. Father every gate opened into my spirit by any means, I cover it with the Blood of Jesus Christ.

5. Dear Lord God, I receive the grace to guard my mouth gate, and every other gateway into my spirit, in the Name of Jesus.

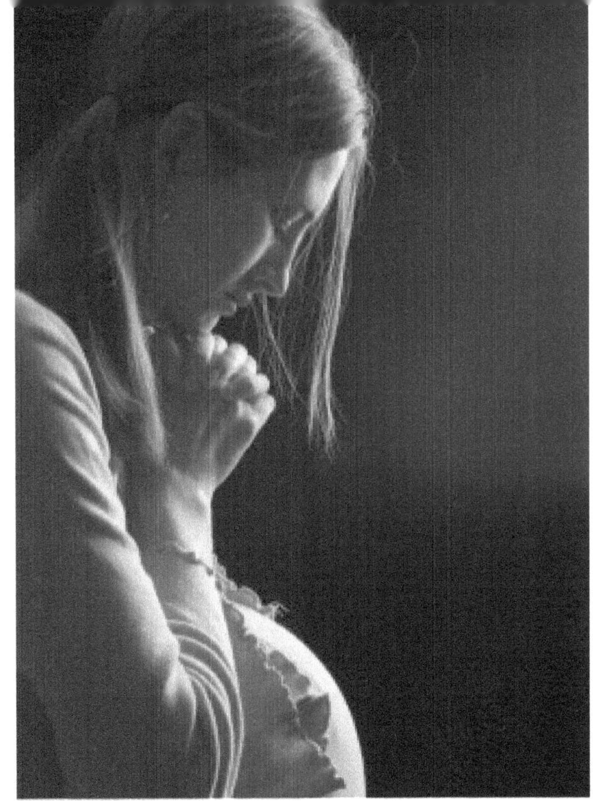

Chapter 7

POLLUTED
GATEWAYS

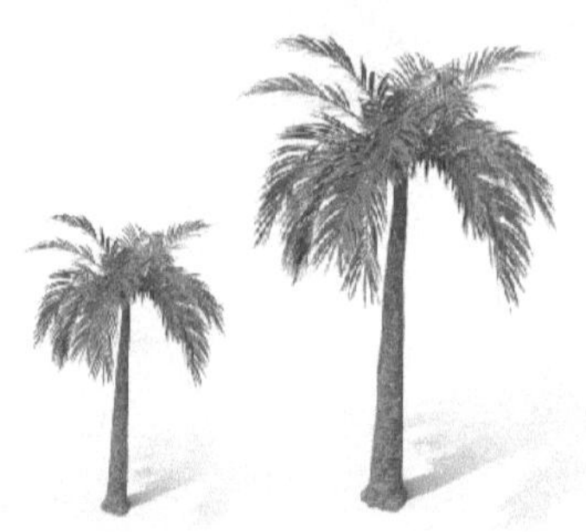

> *Can the fig tree, my brethren, bear olive berries? either a vine, figs? so can no fountain both yield salt water and fresh.*
>
> **James 3:12**

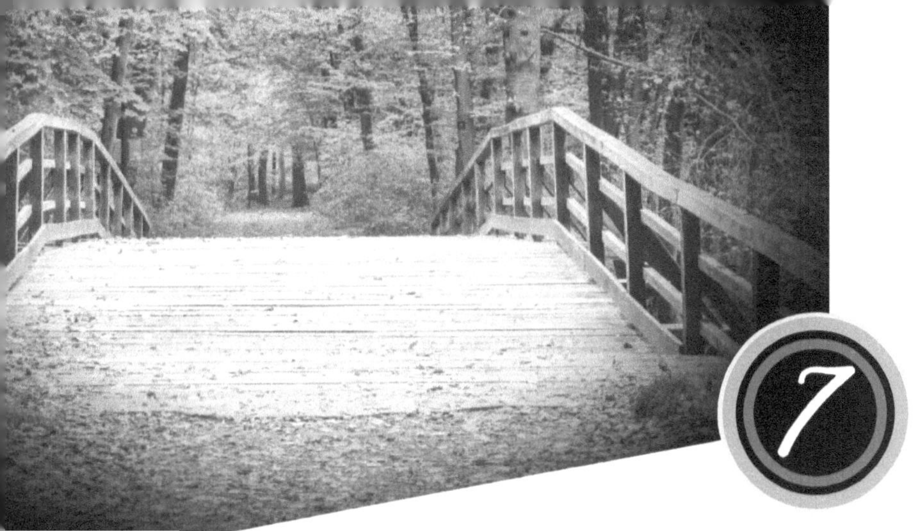

POLLUTED GATEWAYS

> **Who are you to terminate the life of another? Did you create that child?**

In the preceding chapter, we looked at gateways into the womb. It is however, pertinent to reiterate that once the gateway is defiled, the outcome will be dangerous. The reproductive system of a woman is one of the major gateways to the womb. Once this gateway is polluted, the products of such wombs could be dangerously affected.

THE ACT OF PROSTITUTION

Prostitution is the act of providing sexual services to another person in return for payment. God forbids our involvement with prostitutes, because He knows such involvement is detrimental to both men and women.

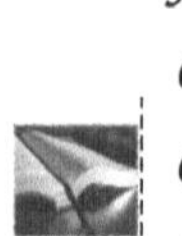

for the lips of an immoral woman drip honey, and her mouth is smoother than oil; but in the end she is bitter as worm wood, sharp as a two-edged sword. Her feet go down to death, her steps lay hold of hell. **Proverbs 5:3-5**

Prostitution not only destroys marriages, families and lives, but destroys the spirit and soul in a way that leads to physical and spiritual death. God's desire is that we stay pure and use our bodies as tools for His use and glory (Romans 6:13).

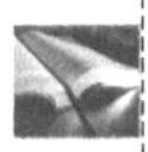 *The body is not for sexual immorality but for the LORD, and the LORD for the body.*
1Corinthians 6:13

A story was told of a young girl – a prostitute who fell into the hands of an occult man. This man wanted a human part for fetish purposes. The man took the girl to a brothel, after having negotiated and agreed on how much the girl would be paid for sexual services rendered. Since the girl was used to having multiple sexual partners, she always carried packets of condoms for her customers.

She brought out a condom and gave to the man, but he rejected it on the grounds that he does not enjoy sex using a condom. The girl told him she was not the only girl with whom he was having sex. She put it to him that he might have been sleeping with other girls, and she did not want to contact HIV/AIDS. The man insisted on doing it without a condom.

While the argument was on, the girl had a device - the rubber cap that women use to protect themselves. It is like a diaphragm. Then she excused herself to use the toilet. She entered the toilet and quickly inserted the device into her body and then came out. The man pleaded with her to have sex unprotected. He gave her a hundred thousand naira (N100,000). The girl accepted, but she had made the insert already.

Then the man went in and pounced on her. As he went in, not even up to ten seconds, the man had ejaculated, and had released everything. As the girl turned, she saw some strange things inching around. She checked closely, alas, they were worms (maggots), and not sperm.

The man quickly picked the worms from the girl's body. But the girl took one, looked at it closely and asked to ease herself. Then she got up, stark-naked, and ran out. She was then screaming, "I am not mad oh! I am not mad! I am not mad! I am not mad!" She ranted to the reception of the hotel.

They were asking her, "What is wrong with you? You are not mad but you are naked."

She said, "An occultic man wanted to use me to do juju."

The idea was that if those maggots entered into her, she would die on the spot, and the man would take what he wanted to take from her. It is quite a recent event. The girl was shouting, "I am not mad! I am not mad!" meanwhile, maggots were inching out of her body, because of one hundred thousand naira.

Can you imagine how that body had been defiled because of the love of money?

What are you introducing into your womb?

Many girls defile their wombs to the extent that when they get married eventually, they will have difficulties getting pregnant. All kinds of complications will arise. *O Lord, let Your mercy prevail over judgment!*

I know of one woman who was indulging in casual sex with multiple partners. She was reckless and preferred money to her future and her God.

Well, eventually, she decided to settle down with one man. And as they became married, she got pregnant. We thought she was fortunate. It was time to bring forth the baby, but she could not give birth. Will Zion get pregnant and not bring forth? No. For her to bring forth the baby became a problem.

They did not only cut her body open to bring out the baby, they had to remove the entire womb. Then they barely managed to stitch it up, because she was bleeding from every part of the body. They did so in order that she would not die. They removed the womb, and brought out a baby girl. This child has been a source of grief to the woman. The child has refused to be tamed.

Since the girl is the only child, the mother has been running up and down to make sure she has the best of education, attention and all of that. The girl is well over thirty years of age. She has attended five different universities, but has not graduated. Her work is to go after men.

So, the woman called me one day and asked, "What do I do?" And I told her, "Your womb was polluted." Even though it was removed, the product of the womb continues to speak. The evil that men do, lives after them. I told her to bring repentance before God in prayer.

Many women made mistakes as young girls; but some were more careless than others were.

When you abort, you have broken a commandment; a serious commandment for that matter.

The blood of the innocent continues to speak against you, and God Himself is not happy with you either, because that child that you aborted has the right to be alive. Yet, you terminated the life of the child.

Who are you to terminate the life of another?

Did you create that child?

Do you know what the child would have become?

Imagine if your mother had aborted you when she was pregnant with you, would you be here?

I know that most women reading this are saying, "Thank God I am not like that." But our daughters! Our daughters! Our children, oh!

You see, no matter how I write, I try to incorporate children. I have a passion for praying for children. I see them, and my heart bleeds when I see what they are doing. You know why I cry for them? Because I am thinking of their tomorrow.

If you eat your tomorrow today, what will you do when the long awaited tomorrow comes?

My mother of blessed memory used to call it, "beautiful nonsense - fine face, rotten bottom." When a man sees such a girl, he will say this is "Miss Nigeria," I must marry her. "Miss Calabar," "Miss Uyo," I must marry her.

When she gets home, she cannot cook. Even to sweep, she cannot, let alone be able to wash her own clothes. Then when she gets pregnant, she becomes a problem to herself and the people around her.

What are we teaching our children? We need to read this hard truth so that we shall be delivered. You may look at it, and say, this woman is too worried about children. It is true. I am really very worried about children. I wish I could stop worrying about them, but I cannot; it is difficult. They are our tomorrow.

Understand this: Your children are your old age support. Do you not know that they are your pension? I am talking about your children. They are the people that are going to cover your nakedness. If they are not standing well today, how will your tomorrow be like?

Tell me, where is your joy as a mother if your children are not successful in life?

I want you to declare that in the evening of your life, you will not be naked. Your children will always bring you joy. Your head will not go down in shame.

The Bible calls children your heritage from the LORD. Imagine a woman like Jochebed, the mother of Moses, Miriam and Aaron. The three children were all prominent in the nation. Will anybody forbid such a thing?

Aaron was the first high priest. Miriam was a prophetess. And Moses was a deliverer. Jochebed was a woman like you and I. If she had a polluted womb, do you think God would have given her those wonderful children?

God is looking for wombs that are pure altars; wombs that are not polluted, and that are usable. Can God use your womb?

Most of the products of the womb become defiled because the gateway is defiled. Most times, our children grow up to be like us.

I have a friend that said to me, "Anything that a snake gives birth to must be long." If you look well, your child does not look like an outsider. He looks like you. If not you, then he resembles your husband.

You must pray for repentance today over the things you did in your prime, which has or can affect the life and future of your children. Pray according to Psalms 25:7 - *"O Lord, do not remember the rebellious sins of my youth. Remember me in the light of Your unfailing love, for You are merciful O Lord."*

We went for prison visitation some years ago. You know, normally the prisoners will not tell their parents the truth; but being a prison pastor myself, when I go, they will say, "Mama, I want to tell you the truth."

There was a young boy in that particular prison, who killed his identical twin brother. He said that a juju priest asked him to kill his twin brother, and bring certain parts from his dismembered body. This was to be used to perform some money rituals for him. So he killed his twin brother and took the parts to the juju priest.

Eventually, the police came and started investigating the incident. There is no way a father or mother would believe that his or her child could kill the other; especially that they were identical twins. Anyone would believe an outsider did it. One could even arrest a husband's relation, uncle, etc. But unfortunately, it was this young man who killed his twin brother.

This boy said that most nights, he was not able to sleep; his late brother's spirit was haunting him. Blood was speaking against him. He was not happy. He said, "Mummy, what do I do? I have confessed my sins, but the thing is still worrying me."

I had to tell him the story of a man called 'David' in the Bible. He asked God to forgive him of his sins, but the consequences were still standing. When David went to sleep with Bathsheba, Uriah's wife, he enjoyed it all right. He killed Uriah. No problem. He was the king. No one dared to ask him. When eventually someone sent of God confronted him, David pleaded for mercy. He said, "God, have mercy upon me."

God said, "I have forgiven you. But someone else will sleep with your wives."

Consequence!

There are consequences.

Take note of this truth.

God can forgive you, but He may not spare you the consequences. The consequences may be standing there, looking at you. There is usually a pay day! You better avoid evil in the first place.

What are you introducing into your womb? Whatsoever a man sows, that he shall reap.

Take a look, for instance, at the Boko Haram people in Northern Nigeria. A good number of them are young men. They did not descend from heaven.

So, what happened?

Let's look at the scenario: Most of them are young boys and girls born out of wedlock. They are street hutchins - also called almajiris. They do not have proper home upbringing, no home discipline and no formal education.

And you know they are offended with the whole world. They are not happy. They say, *"How come people's children are doing well, and we are not doing well? Nobody is showing interest in things that concern us."* Out of frustration, they are easily provoked and they have the tendency to be very violent.

If you go to the Niger Delta where you have violence; I am talking about the riverine areas of Nigeria, there are so many young boys. Most of them are products of sexual immorality. Their mothers had them when they were very young. There was no paternal influence.

If you ask them, "*What is your name?*"

They will say, "*I am bearing my maternal grandfather's name.*"

What are you introducing into your womb? It is what you are introducing into your womb that is causing the trouble in Nigeria and whatever country you come from.

I have shared it in a women conference about a boy that killed his mother. He is still in prison custody today.

What provoked the boy to the point of killing his mother was that a 29-year-old boy was dating his mother. Before her son finally killed her, she had previously married three men at different times. Meanwhile the woman herself was about 56 years old.

The mother of the 29-year-old boy was always crying, "I beg you, leave my child for me." She must have insisted, "I must marry your son." Then, on top of that, her own son was offended that his mother was disgracing them (her children), sleeping around with men.

When the woman slept with a man, he would give all the money in his bank account to her. So, her son became violent and said, "Okay, since you collect money from men, I will be collecting money from you. And make sure you don't ever say 'no' to my request." Unfortunately, the woman had a quarrel with her son about finance. A fight ensued, which led to her death.

The Bible tells me that my body is the temple of the Living God. He says, whosoever destroys the temple shall be destroyed. That means, when you introduce all kinds of rubbish into your body, you bring a curse unto yourself.

Every altar is holy unto the Lord, including your womb. When you burn a strange fire on the altar, the Lord God Almighty who is the consuming fire will release fire upon you.

Look at Aaron's two sons. When they burnt incense with strange fire, the Bible says, fire came. Where did the fire come from?

When you introduce a weird thing into the altar, be prepared for trouble, because you have polluted the gateway. Whatever will come from it may not benefit you.

Take Time Out to Pray

1. O God, let every strange lifestyle flee from my spirit and let the Holy Ghost take control, in the Name of Jesus.

2. My Father, I repent of every unholy or unrighteous acts of immorality or abortion in the past. Let all multiple strongmen operating against me be paralyzed, in the Name of Jesus.

3. Dear Lord, fill me with deep hunger and thirst for righteousness, in the Name of Jesus.

4. Heavenly Father, I decree that my children shall not revel in any manner of life that will pollute their gateways. I confess that my children shall not fish in unprofitable waters.

5. O Lord, release Your tongue of fire upon my life and the life of my children. Burn away all spiritual filthiness present within me, in Jesus' Name.

6. Every anti-repentant spirit in my life, I bind you and cast you out now in Jesus' Name.

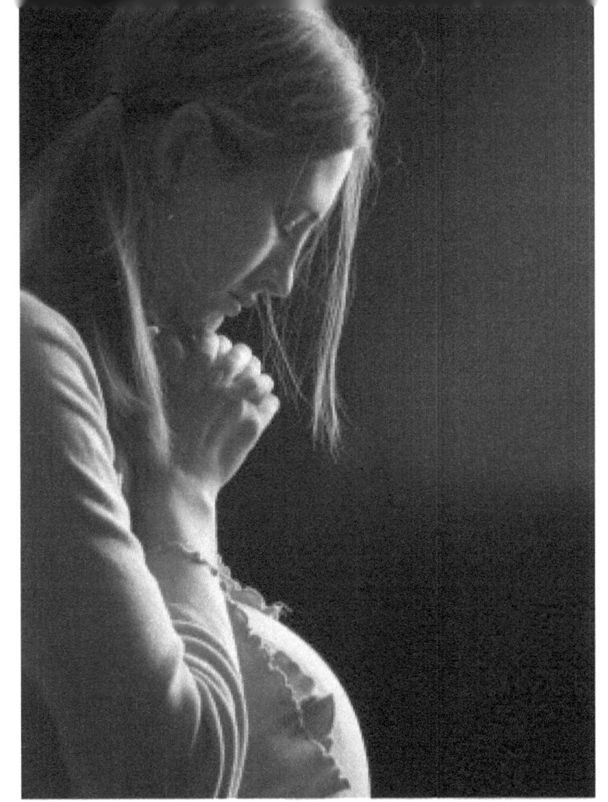

Chapter 8

REBUILDING THE WOMB ALTAR

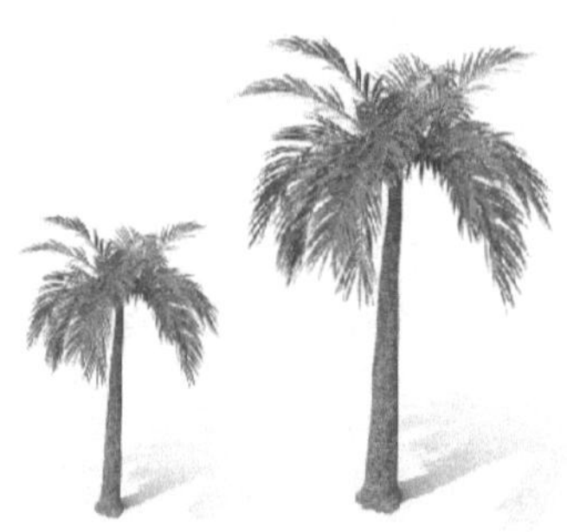

And Elijah said unto all the people, come near unto me. And all the people came near unto him. And he repaired the altar of the LORD that was broken down. And with the stones he built an altar in the name of the LORD: and he made a trench about the altar, as great as would contain two measures of seed.

1Kings 18:30, 32

REBUILDING THE WOMB ALTAR

> " We do not seem to realize that, without God, we cannot accomplish whatever we want to be. "

Israel, under the leadership of Ahab and Jezebel, had desecrated the altar of God by their worship of Baalim. They preferred to worship Baal rather than the eternal God, the Almighty God. They grossly dishonoured God.

Elijah appeared on the scene and proclaimed a drought in the land to show that God utterly disapproved of the nation's idolatrous activities.

This drought threw the nation into famine for a period of three years. For the mercy of God to come down again, Elijah was instructed by God to appear before Ahab. When Elijah appeared before Ahab, he insisted that the 450 prophets of Baal be summoned to a contest to prove whose 'God' answers prayer and erase all forms of doubts.

The prophets called upon Baal to answer them but there was no response, since Baal is an idol, a dead god. But as for Elijah, he had to rebuild the broken down prayer altar. When the stage was fully set, his simple prayer brought down the most dramatic heavenly display the people had ever seen.

In like manner, when an individual has been involved in ungodly activities, he needs to bring a deep repentance before our holy God.

If you were involved in sexual immorality, you defiled the temple of God and so you need to rebuild the altar in the place of prayer.

Of a very serious note is when various atrocious acts have been carried out, that have defiled the womb. Since the womb is an altar, it has to be rebuilt.

Rebuilding the womb altar involves rebuilding the altar of honour. We dishonour God and each other on a regular basis. We want people to see how beautiful we are, how rich we are, how intelligent or brilliant we are, how qualified we are, etc. We do not seem to realize that, without God, we cannot accomplish whatever we want to be.

God said in 1Samuel 2:30b *"those who honour me, I will honour, but those who despise me will be disdained."*

We must learn to honour God with all that we have in life. Many young men and women despise the things of God. They are not spiritually alive. They desecrate the temple of God (their bodies) on the bed of sexual immorality. They do not even like to honour God with their bodies. They feel they have absolute right over their bodies and so can do whatsoever they like. They are morally bankrupt.

Some girls dress in the most obscene ways, exposing the parts of their bodies that ought to be covered. All these are done in the name of fashion.

People indulge in many sinful activities dishonouring God, all in the name of civilization. We destroy the beautiful relationship with God and man because we want to be like the Joneses.

There is, however, a clarion call to come back to God like in the days of Elijah and the prophet of Baal.

And Elijah said unto all the people, come near unto me. And all the people came near him. And he repaired the altar of the lord that was broken down. And with stones he built an altar in the name of the lord; and he made a trench about the altar, as great as would contain two measures of seed.

1Kings 18:30, 32

We live in a nation filled with sin, corruption, sexual immorality, drug, alcohol, violence etc.

Here are some of the excuses for these sinful activities:

Abortion – It is my body and I will do what I want with it. I am not ready to have a child now.

Homosexuality or lesbianism – It is just a way of life. It does not matter, whether I am having sexual intercourse with a same sex partner.

Drugs – It is my life. I will do what I want. It makes me feel cool. It gives me a feeling of belonging.

Alcoholic Drink – I am just a social drinker. After all, the Bible says a little alcohol is good for the belly.

Bribery and Corruption – It is a way of life. Man must learn to be smart. Man must survive. No one can live on just his/her salary alone.

Violence – It is survival of the fittest.

Let me share with you what God's Word says about some of the listed abnormalities as recorded in Isaiah 5:20-25:

> *Woe to those who call evil good and good evil; who put darkness for light and light for darkness; who put bitter for sweet and sweet for bitter.*

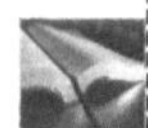

> *Woe to those who are wise in their own eyes and bright in their own sight*

> *Woe to those who are mighty to drink wine,*

and men of strength to mingle strong drink.

Which justify the wicked for a bribe, and take away the righteousness of the righteous from him.

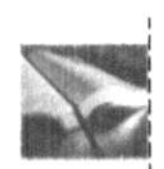

Therefore as the fire devours the stubble, and the flame burns up the chaff, so their root shall be like rottenness, and their blossom shall go up like dust…because they have cast away the law of the lord of hosts; and despised the word of the holy one of Israel.

Therefore is the anger of the lord kindled against his people, and he has stretched out his hand against them, and has stricken them; and the hills trembled and their dead bodies were torn in midst of the streets. For all his anger is not turned away, but his hand is stretched out still.

Taking a close look at the Scripture above, we need to rebuild the broken altar of our hearts.

Now, you may ask, "What is an altar for?"

It is for sacrifice. It is for something to die on.

The next question should be, "What is supposed to die?"

The answer is 'self' – the old rotten sinful self must die so that a brand new self will emerge.

We must bring repentance before God. We must repair the broken down altar of our lives.

This is what the churches need to do. This is what our nation needs to do. The altar of our lives is in a state of gross disrepair.

Elijah had to repair the altar of the Lord that was broken down before he could make a sacrifice for God upon the altar. The Israelites had rejected God, and before they could experience the outpouring of God's power in their lives, the altar had to be repaired and used.

The same holds true for us. If we have rejected God and turned away from him (effectively tearing down the altar), then we need to repair the altar and begin to offer sacrifices again. We must offer the sacrifice of repentance.

Psalm 51:16-17 says, *"you do not delight in sacrifice, or I would bring it; you do not take pleasure in burnt offerings. The sacrifice of God are a broken spirit; a broken and contrite heart, O God, you will not despise."*

When we have neglected the altar of God or we have rejected God, we need to bring a sacrifice of repentance; we need to bring a broken and contrite heart; we need to bring our sorrow for not living like we should.

The second sacrifice is the sacrifice of ourselves. Romans 12:1 says, *"I urge you, brothers, in view of God's mercy, to offer your bodies as a living sacrifice, holy and pleasing to God…this is your spiritual act of worship."*

We need to offer ourselves as a "living sacrifice." Once an animal sacrifice had been offered, that was it. The animal was unable to go on and fulfill any purpose. But as we offer ourselves a living sacrifice, we sacrifice ourselves, our talents, our time, and gifts, our all in all to God.

We cannot risk having a divided loyalty with God. Anytime this happens in the life of an individual, a church or a nation, the altar of worship breaks down and brings about severe hardship and pains.

God is looking for unstoppable worshippers, those who can worship Him in pain, in the wilderness, in spirit and in truth.

God wants us to remove idolatry from our hearts, and homes and give ourselves to pure worship.

From our family to the way we live, we must give Him pre-eminence. God must be First.

God must be honoured always as we allow His Spirit to lead us. We must make God's Words our meat and drink.

Take Time Out to Pray

1. O Lord, I bring repentance before You for every ungodly involvement of my life. I have defiled my body which is Your temple O God. I ask Your forgiveness today, in Jesus' Name.

2. Father I return to You with all my heart like in the days of Elijah. Have mercy on me O God.

3. O God, let my old rotten sinful self die and let a brand new me emerge to glorify You. Let the broken altar of my heart be mended in the Name of Jesus.

4. Father, I receive the grace to rebuild the broken altar in my life in the Name of Jesus.

5. I offer my body today as a "living sacrifice" to You O Lord: My talents, my time, and gifts, my all in all to You O God, in the Name of Jesus.

6. Father help me to experience the outpouring of Your power in my life, in the Name of Jesus.

7. Heavenly Father, please empower me and my seed to stand firm against all the schemes and techniques of the devil to take us back into worldliness, in the Name of Jesus.

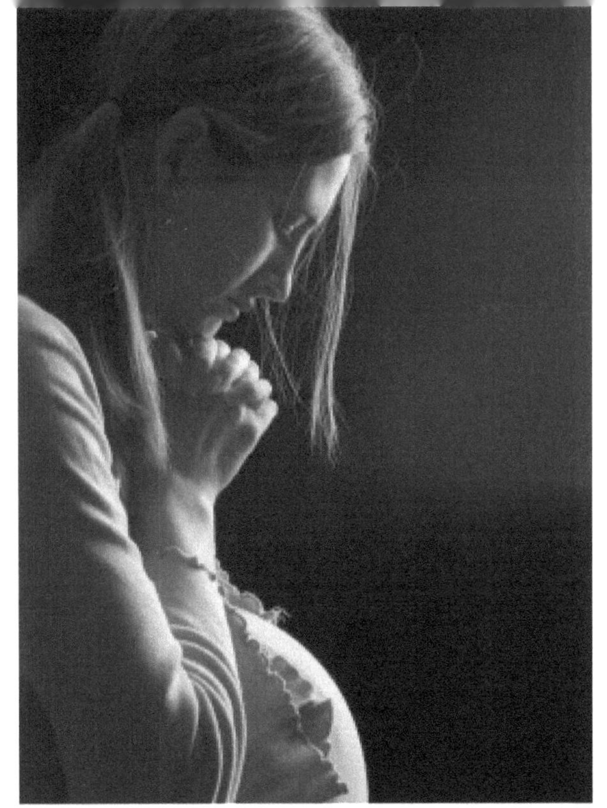

Chapter 9

BIRTH DEFECTS FROM THE WOMB

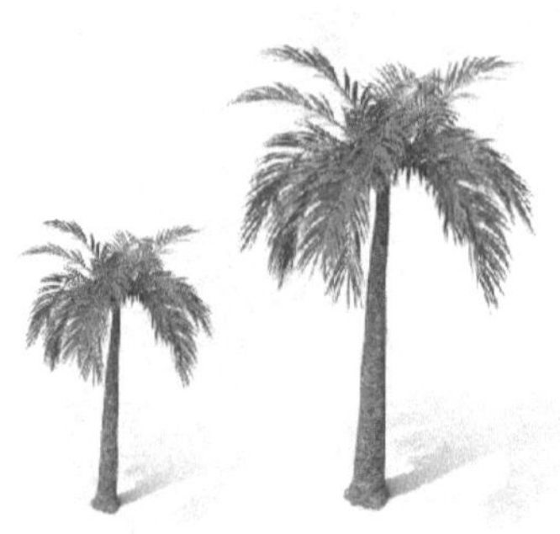

And as Jesus passed by, he saw a man which was blind from his birth.

John 9:1

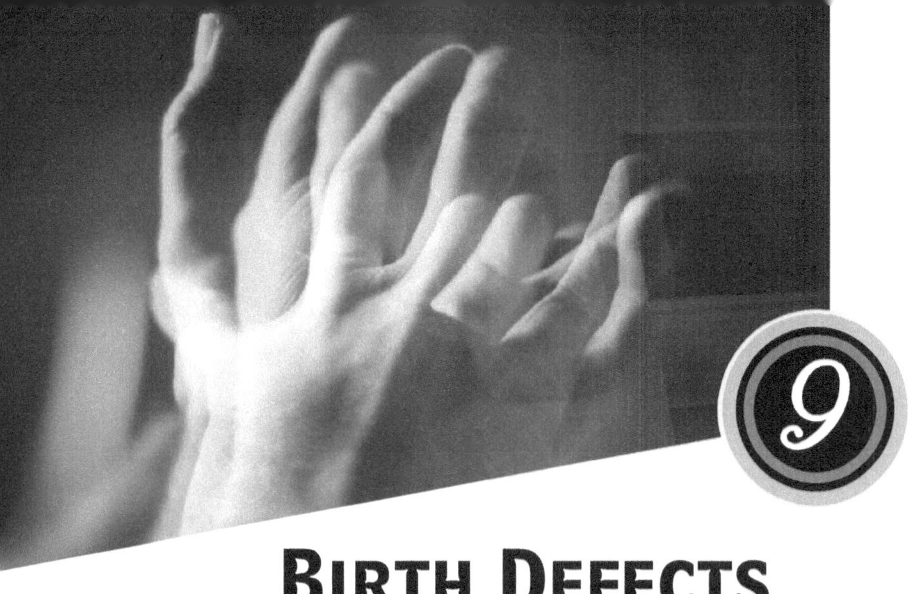

BIRTH DEFECTS FROM THE WOMB

> **Every child is created in God's image, is loved by Him, and has an important purpose in this life.**

Birth defects are structural or functional abnormalities present at birth that cause physical or mental disability. They are the leading causes of death for infants during the first year of life.

Most children are born with one form of birth

defect or the other. A good portion of these happen right from the womb.

Birth defects might be structural or functional:

Structural birth defects are related to a problem with body parts such as heart defects and abnormal limbs.

Functional birth defects are related to a problem with how a body part or body system works. These problems often lead to developmental disabilities and can include things such as nervous system or brain problems, sensory problems, metabolic disorders, and degenerative disorders.

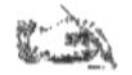 ## THE MAN BORN BLIND

In John 9:1 the Bible talks about a man with a noticeable birth defect: "*And as Jesus passed by, he saw a man which was **blind from his birth**.*"

This implies that the man was blind right from the womb. Why this man was born blind could be understood from Jesus' answer to His disciples' question:

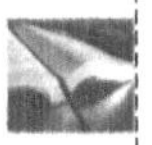 *Master, who did sin, this man, or his parents, that he was born blind?"* (John 9:2).

Jesus said, *"Neither hath this man sinned, nor his parents: but that the works of God should be made manifest in him"* (John 9:3).

Jesus' answer to His disciples showed that SIN can be a major cause of some form of defect or the other in children as we have already seen in earlier chapters of this book.

Tainted by the sin that began with Adam and Eve in the Garden of Eden, all humanity to follow has been under the curse of sin in this world. Though Jesus offers a cure to sin through belief in His Name.

The consequences of fallen humanity

continue to be displayed in a variety of ways, including in the youngest members of society.

Howbeit, the blindness of this person was not occasioned by any sin of his own, nor of his parents, but had happened in the ordinary course of Divine providence.

His case eventually became the instrument of salvation to his soul, edification to others, and glory to GOD.

THE MAN BORN LAME

Another person we find with a birth defect is the lame man at the Gate called Beautiful.

Acts 3:2 says, *"And a certain man lame from his mother's womb was carried, whom they laid daily at the gate of the temple which is called Beautiful, to ask alms of them that entered into the temple;"*

Again, like the blind man, this man was lame

right from the womb. The Bible does not say anything about the cause of his condition here, and we should neither assume nor claim to know it. This defect was there right from the womb.

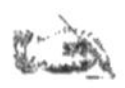

CRIPPLED FROM THE WOMB

Another account of a man that was wounded from his mother's womb is found in Acts 14:8:

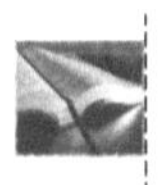

And there sat a certain man at Lystra, impotent in his feet, being a cripple from his mother's womb, who never had walked:

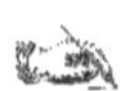

BUT WHY?

At this point, you might want to ask, why does God allow birth defects in the first place? This question is a tough one to handle, especially for parents who have children with disabilities.

From the foregoing, however, it is clear from the words of Jesus that birth defects might serve as part of God's plan for some people's life. It is extremely difficult, though, as humans, to accept or understand this. Nevertheless, since we often simply do not know the specific reasons God allows a child to have a birth defect, we can know every child is created in God's image, is loved by Him, and has an important purpose in this life.

GOD MAY DO IT

God sometimes orchestrates a wounded womb. One case in point can be seen as recorded in Hosea 9:11-17:

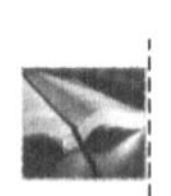

> *As for Ephraim, their glory shall fly away like a bird, from the birth, and from the womb, and from the conception. Though they bring up their children, yet will I bereave them, that there shall not be a man left: yea, woe also to*

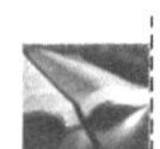

them when I depart from them! Ephraim, as I saw Tyrus, is planted in a pleasant place: but Ephraim shall bring forth his children to the murderer. Give them, O LORD: what wilt thou give? give them a miscarrying womb and dry breasts. All their wickedness is in Gilgal: for there I hated them: for the wickedness of their doings I will drive them out of mine house, I will love them no more: all their princes are revolters. Ephraim is smitten, their root is dried up, they shall bear no fruit: yea, though they bring forth, yet will I slay even the beloved fruit of their womb. My God will cast them away, because they did not hearken unto him: and they shall be wanderers among the nations.

Ephraim's dedication to idol worship and acts of immorality earned the Judgement of God. All the glory of the past would vanish. Women would be struck barren. And the children they were rearing would live with sorrow and death.

Ephraim exchanged their glory for abomination. They were given the sentence:

"No birth, no pregnancy, and no conception."

The future generation would not survive. What is the implication of this? Simple: A nation that does not procreate will fall into ruin, and this is what God was saying.

Can you imagine someone losing his glory right from his mother's womb? The person is enveloped in reproach and misery.

Can you imagine how many people have lost their glory right from the womb? How can a person in that class amount to anything near greatness in life? Such a person is already destined to be a failure or a nonentity.

The womb of a woman is the gateway to life. When the womb is tampered with, the seed planted inside can be negatively affected. The product of a wounded womb could give rise to a birth defect or destiny distortion.

I pray for you today, that your womb will not produce a crippled child (whether physically or spiritually), in Jesus' Name. Please pray a little before proceeding:

1. I decree and declare that my children are released from the grip of any problem, transfered into their life from the womb in the Name of Jesus.

2. I disconnect my children from every collective evil covenant in the Name Jesus.

3. Any rod of the wicked rising up against my family line, be rendered impotent in Jesus' Name.

4. I refuse to drink from the fountain of sorrow in Jesus' Name.

5. I dissociate myself and my family members from every evil covenant and generational curses in the Name of Jesus.

Besides some birth defects being the act of God, there are teratogens that are inimical to the foetus in the womb.

Teratogens are substances or other factors that can cause congenital abnormalities or birth defects.

Usually, these abnormalities arise in the third to eighth weeks of pregnancy, when the major organ systems are forming.

Examples of teratogens include certain chemicals, medications, and infections, or other diseases in the mother.

CHEMICALS AND MEDICATIONS

It is difficult to determine whether a particular chemical or medication causes congenital abnormalities. This is because many women take medications during pregnancy, and most studies have to rely on the mother's memory of what she took while she was pregnant.

One notable exception is ***thalidomide***, a medication used to treat morning sickness, which was found in the 1960s to cause total or partial absence of the arms or legs in babies.

Some other medications known to cause congenital abnormalities of the foetus are as follows:

1. ***Aminopterin.*** This is a drug that is used to treat cancerous tumours. Aminopterin blocks folic acid, and folic acid is important for production of DNA and cell growth.

2. Some ***anti-epileptic drugs*** are associated with a wide array of birth defects, such as cardiovascular abnormalities, cleft palate, and microcephaly, which is a condition where the brain is too small.

3. *Warfarin,* a blood-thinning drug.

4. Some types of *tranquilizers*, such as *phenothiazine* and *lithium*, are thought to be teratogens.

Similarly, drugs used to treat anxiety, such as *diazepam*, are linked with congenital abnormalities such as cleft lip or palate.

ALCOHOL, SMOKING, AND OTHER DRUGS

Alcohol

Alcohol use is a well-known cause of congenital abnormalities during pregnancy. Even moderate amounts of alcohol in pregnancy can cause developmental problems in the unborn baby.

Abnormalities caused by alcohol in pregnancy include deformities of the face, arms, and legs, heart conditions, mental retardation, and fetal growth restriction. However, these conditions are not very common. More frequently, children born to women who drink heavily during pregnancy, may have problems with thinking and remembering and behavioural issues.

The abnormalities and other problems caused by alcohol use in pregnancy are referred to as *Fetal Alcohol Spectrum Disorder*.

Cigarette Smoking

Cigarette smoking is linked with fetal growth restriction and premature birth. Smoking may also cause problems with the development of the brain, cardiovascular system, and respiratory system. This is true whether the mother smokes herself or is exposed to second-hand smoke.

Babies exposed to cigarette smoke during pregnancy may also be born with an increased startle reflex, tremor, or other problems. The effects of cigarette smoke on the unborn baby increase with how much the mother smokes, as well as the length of time she has been smoking.

Marijuana

Exposure to *marijuana* during pregnancy may result in low birth weight, intracranial bleeding, jitteriness, low blood sugar, low levels of calcium in the blood, or an infection of the blood called sepsis.

The use of marijuana in pregnancy can cause other problems in the baby, such as poor feeding, irritability, and rapid breathing.

Amphetamines

Amphetamines, also called "speed," stimulate the central nervous system.

Prenatal use of these drugs is associated with premature birth, low birth weight, or intracranial bleeding.

Opioids

The use of **opioid drugs**, such as **heroin** or **methadone**, during pregnancy can lead to fetal growth restriction, premature birth, and low birth weight.

Cocaine

Cocaine use is known to cause numerous problems during pregnancy. These include miscarriage, fetal growth restriction, and problems with the development of the urinary system or genital tract. The use of cocaine can lead to microcephaly, where the brain is too small.

Children of mothers who used cocaine

during pregnancy are also more prone to developing neurobehavioural problems.

Cocaine use during pregnancy has been associated with a higher risk of a serious problem with the placenta, called <u>placental abruption</u>.

Prenatal use of cocaine may also cause increased startling, jitteriness, and excessive sucking in the newborn baby.

The use of all the aforementioned types of drugs during pregnancy can also lead to a condition called ***neonatal abstinence syndrome***, where the baby experiences withdrawal.

When a woman is pregnant and takes one of these drugs, her baby can become addicted. Once born, the baby is still dependent on the drug. Since the drug is no longer available, the baby experiences withdrawal.

X-rays

X-rays can cause problems with fetal development, such as spina bifida, cleft palate, blindness, abnormalities of the arms and legs, or microcephaly, which is a condition where the brain is too small.

The type of abnormality that develops depends on the dose of X-ray radiation the pregnant woman receives, and how far along the pregnancy is.

Radiation and chemotherapy, which are used to treat cancer, are also associated with congenital abnormalities.

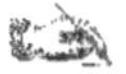

MATERNAL CONDITIONS

A number of chronic illnesses in the mother are linked with an increased risk of congenital abnormalities, fetal growth restriction, or certain diseases in the unborn baby. The chickenpox virus, for instance, is a risk to women who have not already had chickenpox, or who have not been properly vaccinated against that disease.

In some maternal conditions, the risk lies with the drugs used for treatment, rather than the illness itself. It is important to get these conditions under control before becoming pregnant. In some cases, a change in treatment may be needed before pregnancy begins.

From all these, we can see that there are preventable forms of birth defects.

If a mother is careless in some way, and her child is born with a certain birth defect, it is all her fault.

This is very important, so that people do not continue to base every result or outcome on the supernatural.

Many issues can be prevented by avoiding the man-made causes. No woman should be ignorant of these practices that can be harmful to the growth of the baby in her womb.

Take Time Out to Pray

1. Father, I stand against any birth defect in my babies and claim perfection for them, in the Name of Jesus.

2. I pray for the members of my family today. I claim proper growth and development for the babies in the womb of pregnant women. I declare safety for them during childbirth in Jesus' Name.

3. Any abnormality in my organs of conception, receive
Divine correction in the Name of Jesus.

4. Anything on my way to the miracle of supernatural conception and birth, clear away by the Blood of Jesus.

5. Thou creative power of God, move in my womb by Your fire, in the Name of Jesus.

6. Every strong man supervising my womb to arrest my babies, expire in the Name of Jesus.

7. I declare that every disease and germ should die now in Jesus' Name. Nothing I take into my body through the mouth shall harm me or my baby. I look forward to rearing my children after birth, and none shall be defective in Jesus' Name.

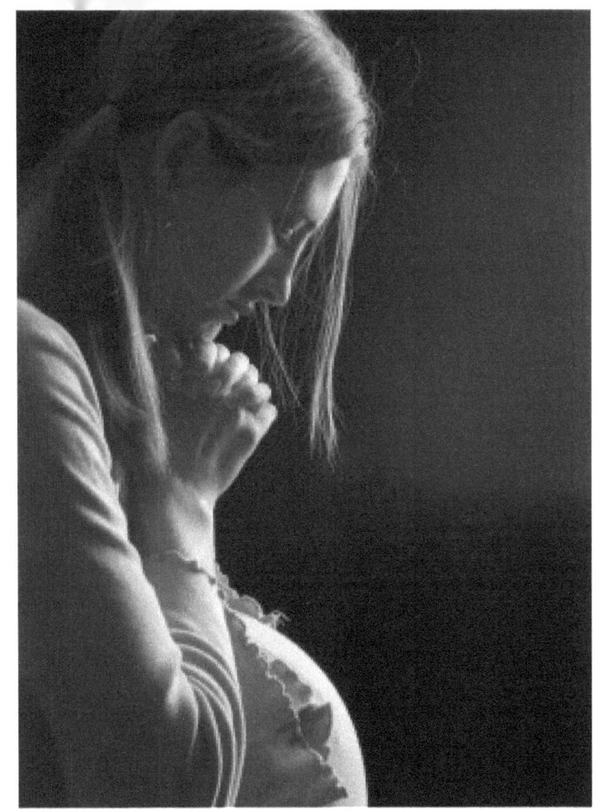

Chapter 10

STAYING PURE

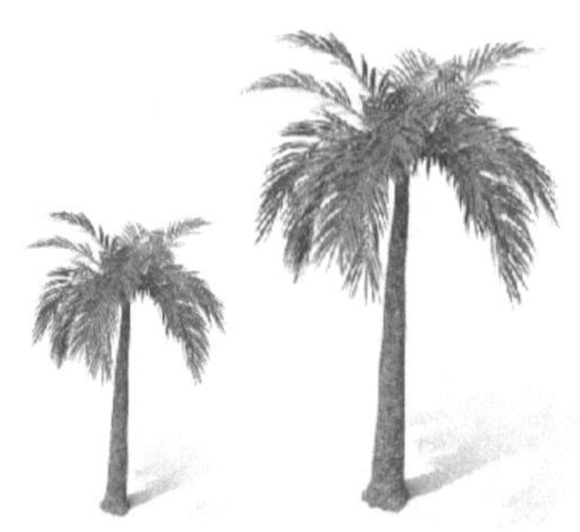

For if after they have escaped the pollutions of the world through the knowledge of the Lord and Savior Jesus Christ, they are again entangled therein, and overcome, the latter end is worse with them than the beginning ...

2 Peter 2:20

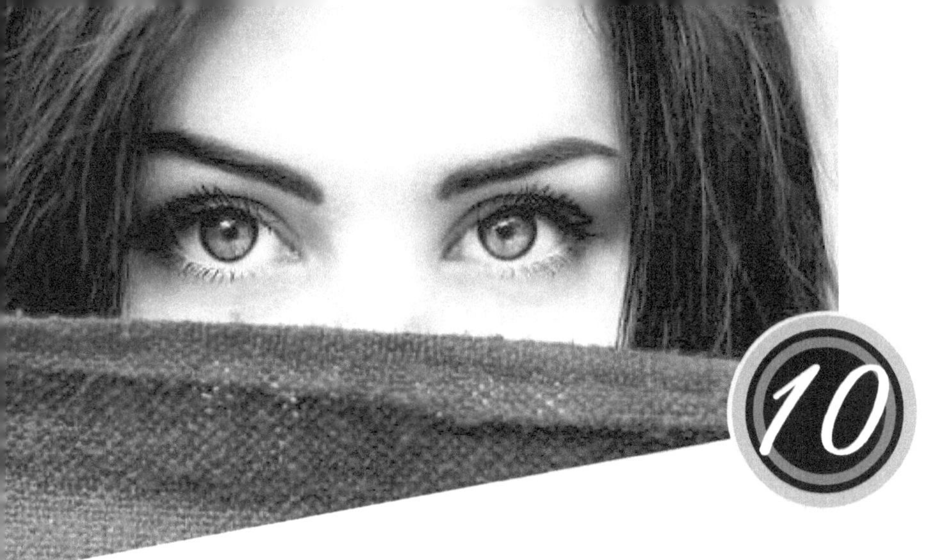

STAYING PURE

> " *It is one thing to be set free from the grievous grip of the past, and another thing to stand firm in the principles of God's Word.* "

I'll love to conclude this wonderful book with a word on staying pure and unpolluted. That is, maintaining what God has done in your life and moving from glory to glory every passing day.

Going back into any form of pollution is not

an option at this point. The Apostle Peter says it is better to have never known the way of righteousness, than to turn back from it to the old filthiness. He compares people who do that to dogs and swine.

Many people receive God's mercy for their filthy old life, but few are able to show appreciation for what He has done by staying pure, unpolluted and perpetually connected to His grace. Many soon relapse into sin and get entangled afresh. Of such, the Apostle Peter says *"the latter end is worse with them than the beginning."*

It is one thing to be set free from the grievous grip of the past and another thing to stand firm in the principles of God's Word.

The Apostle Paul writing to the Galatians said, *"Stand fast therefore in the liberty wherewith Christ hath made us free, and be not entangled again with the yoke of bondage"* (Galatians 5:1).

Now that the Lord has forgiven and purged you from every pollution of your life, do not allow the world and its lusts to pull you back into sin. Stand fast in the faith and use the power that the Lord has given you both to submit yourself to Him and resist the devil, and he will flee from you (James 4:7).

It is easy to relapse into the same old ways if you do not fill your heart with the Word of God; if you do not pray; and if you do not keep your mind centered and stayed on the Lord. On the other hand, when you make a decision to be set apart from the world and live in holiness and integrity, you unlock the supernatural!

It is important you understand that when the enemy is disgraced out of your life by the power of God, he keeps coming back to see if there is an opening.

Don't let him come back and find you empty!

Don't let him come back and find that you have not filled your life with the Word of God, lest he takes advantage of you.

If you provide a loophole for the enemy to access your life, sooner or later you will find yourself again, doing things that you never thought you would. You will find yourself taking pleasure in things you never thought you would. May that never be your experience.

The truth is, what you spend your time doing and what you feed on regularly can affect you in no little measure.

If you spend most of your time watching secular television, listening to secular music, watching the negative news, and hanging out with unbelievers — you will very unlikely have any meaningful spiritual growth.

If you must keep your womb unpolluted, you need to dissociate from many things, including old friends and acquaintances that see your decision to live for God as unfashionable. You can't maintain such friendships and walk with God.

The story is told of a lady who genuinely gave her life to Jesus Christ and walked out of her past sinful life. One day, her former boyfriend (sin partner) came into town and gave her a call. She told him she was a changed person and no longer engaged in such immoral affairs.

The young man seemed fairly excited at the news and told her he needed to see her and hear more about her new life. They agreed on a time to meet. That meeting, however, revived old sinful passions and led to another immoral affair. She returned with deep pains and regrets.

Beloved, the devil hasn't changed. He is the same old devil and knows how to tempt each person to sin from their weakest points. Don't create that opportunity by maintaining old sinful ties.

The Bible warns us again and again that there should be a definite line drawn between us and worldly friends.

In this world, sexual sin, violence, foul language and drunkenness are celebrated, while morality and Christian values are laughed at.

That's why 2Corinthians 6:14-15,17-18 (NLT) says, *"Don't team up with those who are unbelievers. How can righteousness be a partner with wickedness? How can light live with darkness? What harmony can there be between Christ and the devil? How can a believer be a partner with an unbeliever? Therefore, come out from among unbelievers, and separate yourselves from them, says the Lord. Don't touch their filthy things, and I will welcome you. And I will be your Father, and you will be my sons and daughters, says the Lord Almighty."*

God does not want to find us in intimate relationship with people who deride His ways or choose to live in ungodliness.

If you can't convince such people to join you and serve your God, yet keep up with them intimately, they'll surely get you on their side.

The Apostle James said, *"If you want to be a friend of the world, you make yourself an enemy of God"* (James 4:4). That is the simple truth. If you want to continue with friends that keep drawing you backward and polluting your relationship with God, you make yourself an enemy of God.

You have to make the choice to keep yourself pure and your womb unpolluted. Yes, you will be tempted in many ways to do what you wouldn't want to do, but you must make the choice to 'flee' from sin. The Apostle Paul said to young Timothy, "Flee the evil desires..." – 2Timothy 2:22 (NIV).

It is your job to flee. It is your job to keep yourself pure. It is your job to straighten out things that are displeasing to God in your life. It is your job to cleanse yourself daily. 2Corinthians 7:1 says, "Let us cleanse ourselves..." So, the responsibility is yours, not God's.

When your flesh rises up to pressure you to displease God, the Bible says to crucify it (Galatians 5:24). You no longer have to let your flesh live the way it wants to live. Crucify it. When it wants to do or say things it shouldn't, you have to stand your ground and glorify God in your body.

Watch out against everything that is capable of pulling you back into the same old rut. Put on extra caution as a garment wherever you find yourself. Even if you are actively involved in service to God in a Church, I must tell you that adultery, fornication and every kind of sexual immorality is in epidemic proportions in the Church.

You may be very disappointed to see that the people you look up to, can be the ones pressuring you into deadly sinful traps. But you must take a bold stand against satan's work in order to stay unpolluted.

Don't entertain it. Don't consider it. Don't have lunch with it. Don't think twice about it. Flee!

Choose to obey the Word of God. Separate yourself to God. Order your conduct according to the Word of God and the promptings of the Holy Spirit. This will stand you out and distinguish you.

Many people are born again, but they never disconnect from their old lives. They never spend enough time reading God's Word, hearing from God, praying, or learning how to listen to the Holy Spirit within them. As a result, they keep relapsing into the same old sin and eventually get entangled in things that pollute their womb altar and crumble their destiny.

You will keep yourself on God's side by continually putting His Word in your eyes, in your ears, day by day, letting God speak to you, listening to His correction and instruction, and letting His Word prosper your soul.

May God give you the grace to stay pure and keep moving higher in your relationship with the Master. Amen!

Take Time Out to Pray

1. Father I receive grace never to return to the past in the Name of Jesus.

2. Lord help me to stand in the liberty wherewith Christ made me free. May I not be entangled anymore with the yoke of bondage.

3. O God I present myself before You and ask that you do not allow me to be a victim of the deceptions of the enemy of their soul.

4. Heavenly Father please open my eyes and ears in the spirit to the tricks and schemes of the enemy. Help me to stand fast in you Lord and keep my eyes completely fixed on you.

5. O God help please keep Your fire burning in my heart and keep me filled with the desire to seek Your face. Keep me filled with the determination to know You Lord and to know You more and more.

6. Fill me dear Lord with Your precious Holy Spirit and give me the boldness to be a witness to others of Your goodness, mercy, and grace.

7. Let the words of my mouth and the meditations of my heart be acceptable in Your sight Father God.

8. Thank You Father for being my strength. Thank You for being my redeemer. Thank You Father for being my strong tower. Thank You for being my Deliverer, my Provider, and my Peace, in Jesus' Name I pray. Amen.

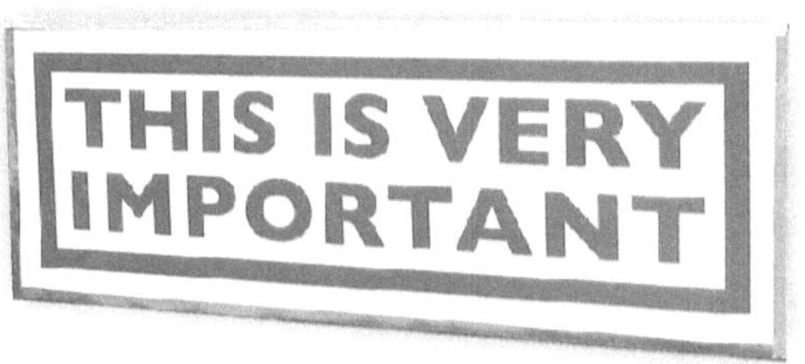

Beloved, you need to surrender your life to the Lordship of Jesus Christ by accepting His sacrificial death on Calvary for you or you need to re-dedicate your life to Jesus Christ.

Pray this prayer with me:

Lord Jesus, I come before You today to surrender my life completely to you. I have lived a self-centred life that is far separated from God, I have had priorities that are not eternity-centred, I have always lived in rebellion, disobedience, and sin up till now.

Lord, I am sorry for the way that I have lived and I ask for your forgiveness and mercy. Lord, please cleanse my sins by your blood and take your place of leadership and rulership in my life.

Fill my heart Lord with the right desires and priorities. Deliver me from the vanity and fantasies of this world.

Give me the grace to say no to sin and compromise. Give me the grace to live in righteousness and represent you well in my world.

Help me to escape the tragedy of eternity in hell. Help me Lord to make heaven at the end of my journey on earth. Help me Lord to live both in the consciousness of your presence and of eternity. Continuously reveal to me everything that would make me unworthy of Heaven.

Thank you Lord for hearing and answering me in Jesus' Name I pray, Amen.

If you have prayed this prayer, please do the following:

1. Send us your name, phone number, and contact address by email: *edewede21@yahoo.com* or by phone: *+234 803 676 9278*

2. Become serious with God by identifying with a righteousness and eternity-conscious church.

3. Study your Bible daily to receive a word from God.

4. Speak to God daily in prayer and let Him know your feelings and challenges.

5. Disconnect from every wrong association. Don't follow them to hell if they won't follow you to Heaven.

6. Speak to others about God. Share your testimony of transformed life. Be instrumental in assisting someone to escape hell.

7. Repent promptly. Do not sleep over unconfessed sins. Apply the blood over your soul for cleansing continuously. Live eternity ready.

The Lord bless you.

Other Books by
Dr Augusta Ogbene

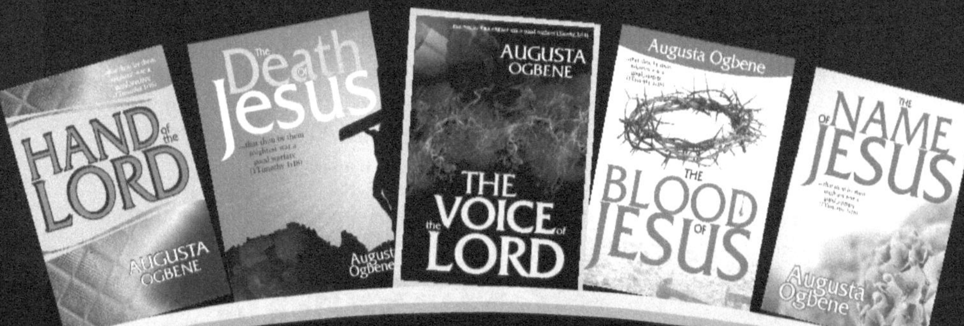

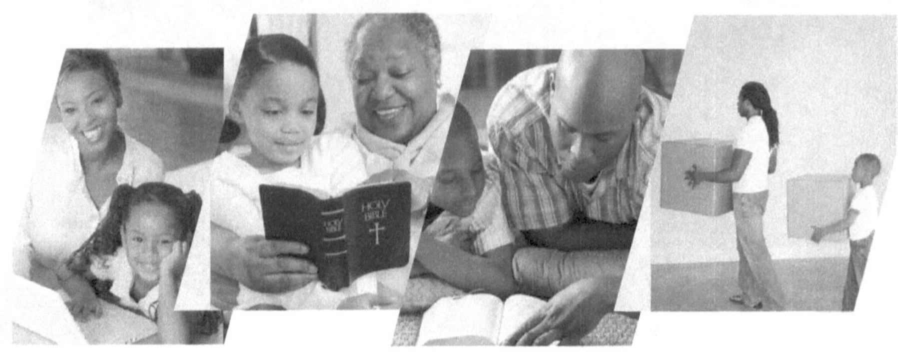

what is your greatest Desire? for your children

'**Y**ES! You want your children to know the Lord and to walk in His ways. You want them to be useful in the hands of God, and to be a blessing to their generation.

■ You want your children to surpass your achievements in life. You want them to be exceptional, extraordinary, and outstanding. You want them to be history makers, world changers, trend setters and trail blazers.

■ You want your children to understand what God wants them to accomplish with their life on earth early enough.

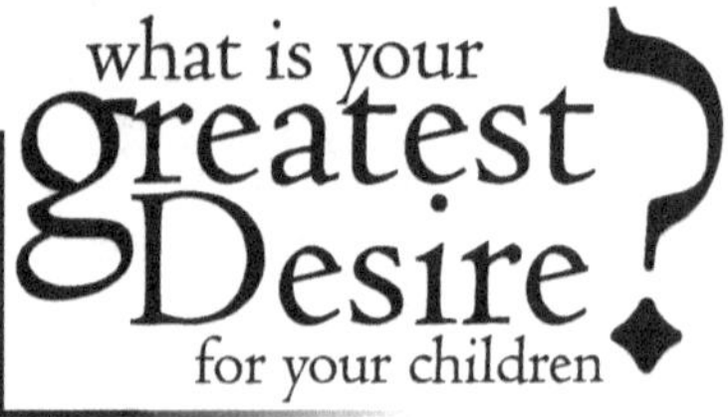

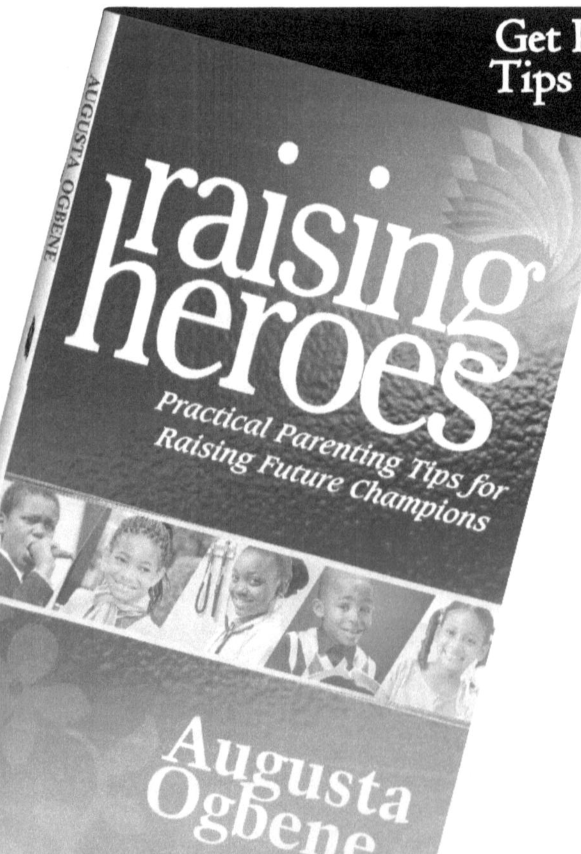

In this book, Dr. Augusta shares Word-proven practical steps to bringing out the hidden hero in your children. Now you have in your hands the tool to help your children fulfill God's unchanging purpose for their lives.

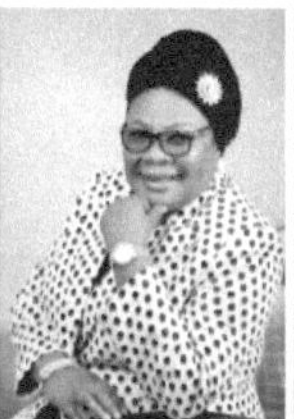

More Books By
DR AUGUSTA OGBENE

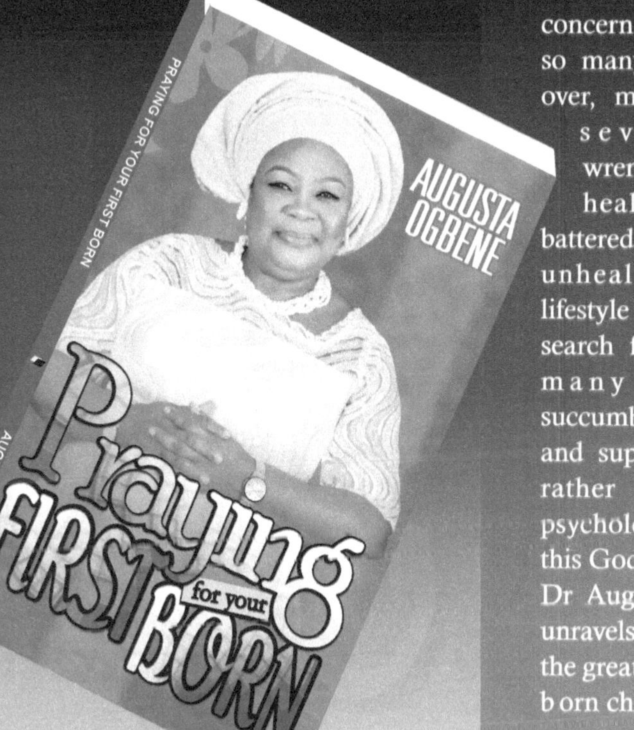

The first born child is the concern of many a parent. In so many homes the world over, marriages have been severed, hearts wrenched, money lost, healthy relationships battered, etc., because of the unhealthy or wayward lifestyle of a first born. In search for lasting solution, many parents have succumbed to religious lies and superstitions that have rather left the situation psychologically worse. In this God-sent book however, Dr Augusta breaks the ice, unravels hidden truths about the greatness inherent in first b orn children and shows the way to get them to manifest it!

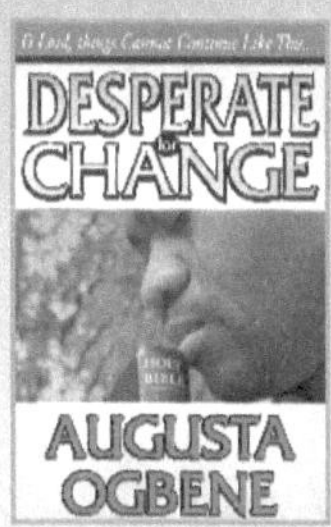

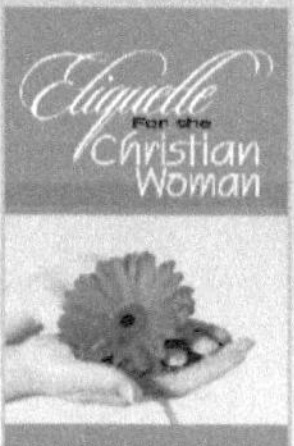

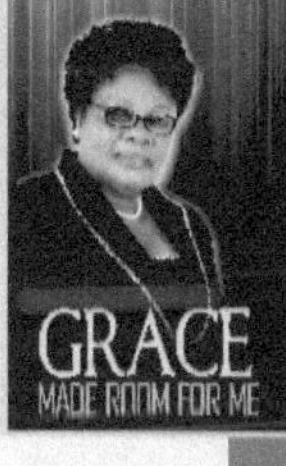

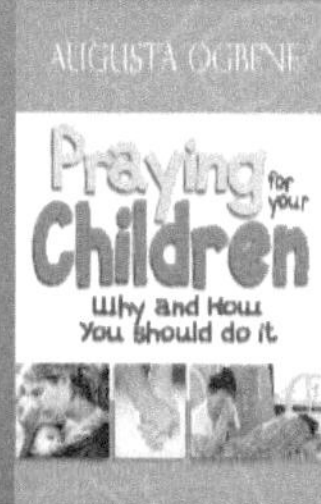

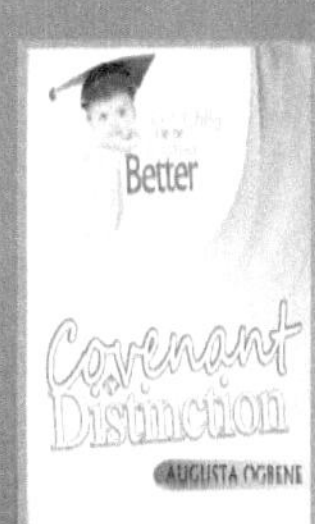

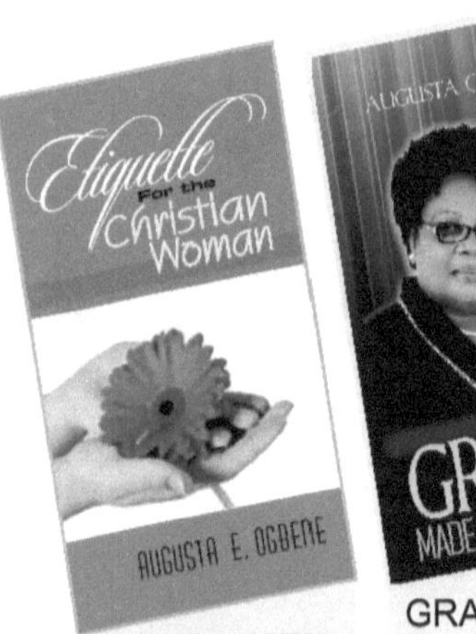

ETIQUETTE FOR THE CHRISTIAN WOMAN

Etiquette for the Christian Woman is an all round book specially designed for the all round building and rebuilding of the Christian woman. Dr Augusta here focuses on the beauty of the whole woman; beauty that works from the inside out. Written in a simple, straight forward and balanced style, the book takes care of the appearance, conduct, comportment, body care, character and lifestyle of the Christian woman at home and in public.

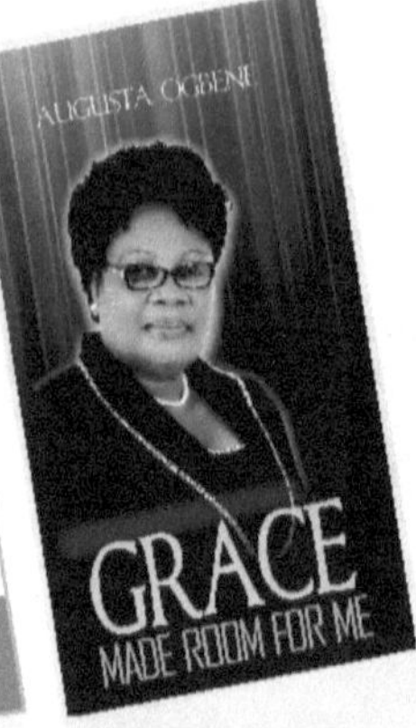

GRACE MADE ROOM FOR ME

It is by God's grace that we find favour with God and man. Most of the time people don't even know why they like us, accept us, trust us, approve of us over others. They just do because God shines His light of grace upon us and gives us favour. Dr Augusta in this little impact full book, shares the story of grace in the life of Ruth. Nothing else but grace made room for her in a strange land. Nothing else but grace will make room for you in this life. Read this book, understand it, live it.

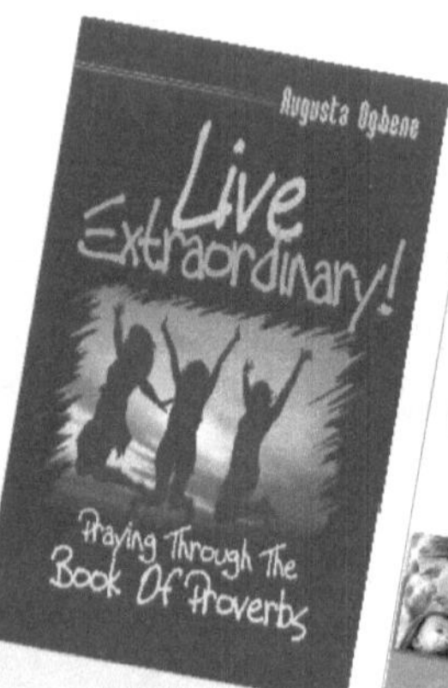

LIVE EXTRA-ORDINARY!

God releases His power according to the authority of His Word which you declare through prayers. Everything that can cause failure to man spiritually, physically, mentally, socially, or financially can get solved through the Book of Proverbs. A combination of the power of the Word and the power of prayer can transform any life, including yours. Praying through the Book of Proverbs will influence every aspect of your life and that of the people around you. Get ready to live extraordinary!

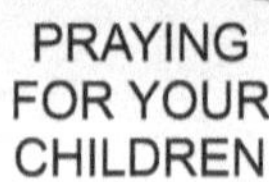

PRAYING FOR YOUR CHILDREN

It is indeed, very difficult and dangerous to raise up children without adequate spiritual cover over them, especially that there is such overwhelming deluge of ungodliness in the rank and file of the society in which they grow. Until parents can learn to take their children to God on their knees, they may watch with dismay, the ungodly and strange habits the children may exhibit now and in their future lives. This book will help parents to resist in prayer, the spirit of this age from manifesting in the life of their children.

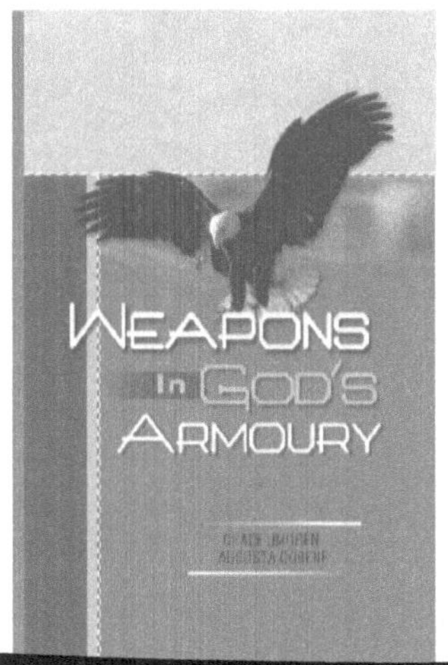

FIGHT WITH GOD'S WEAPONS!

We are involved in Spiritual Warfare daily. The warfare is not against flesh and blood but against principalities and powers, against spiritual wickedness in the high places of the world. To be ignorant that we are fighting a spiritual battle daily is to be victims of the devil. To be ignorant of the weapons that the Lord has provided for us and how to make effective use of them is to put our destiny in the hands of the enemy to manipulate. This book is created for you to defeat your one greatest enemy, Satan (the devil).If you really desire to know the weapons that God has provided for you to have constant victory, read this book.

BE ALL YOU SHOULD BE!

DAILY CAPSULES helps you draw near to God through personal knowledge of His Word and also helps you make your faith active by declaring His promises over your life. Meditating over His Word and declaring it over your life will change the way you think, the way you talk, the way you act, and the way God would move in and through your life. God wants you to think, talk, and act like He means what He says!

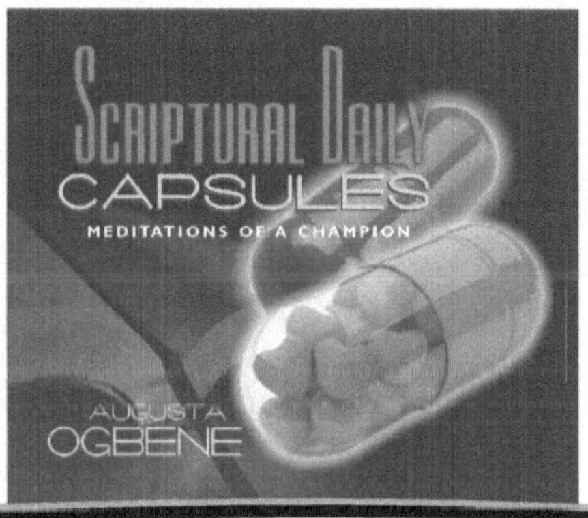

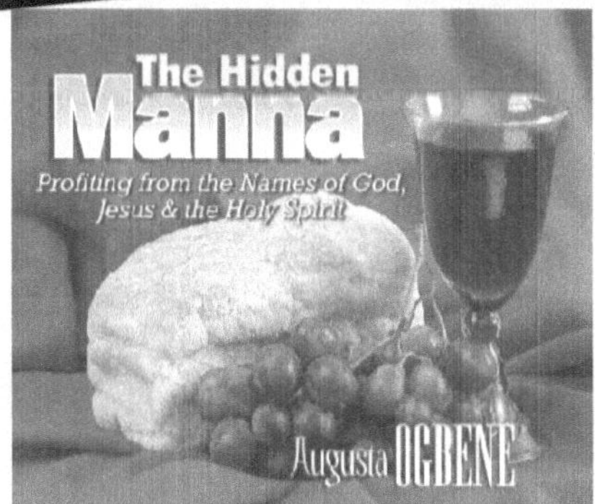

THERE IS POWER IN HIS NAME

God's Name is a strong tower for us. In His Name we may take rest when we are weary and take refuge when we are pursued. In His Name we may be lifted up above our enemies and fortified against them. There is enough in God. The wealth laid up in His Name is enough to enrich us. The strength in His Name is enough to protect us. The Hidden Manna brings to your spirit a revelation of the power in the Names of God, of the Lord Jesus Christ, and of the Holy Spirit.

Index

A

Index

dangerous, 145
Daniel, 98
darkness, 107, 172, 212
dating, 161
David, 31, 44, 86, 157-158
deadly, 215
decent, 109
declaration, 114
decree, 163, 191
dedication, 88, 189
defect, 184-188, 191, 200,
defile, 58, 150
deformities, 194
degenerative, 184
delay, 63
delicate, 106
deliverance, 122
demonic, 57, 125
depth, 12
deride, 213
descendants, 34, 103, 140
desecrate, 170
desire, 56, 63, 111, 131,
desolate, 33
despise, 169-170, 175
destiny, 1, 3, 14, 20, 33,
56, 62-63, 83, 85, 88, 91-92, 108, 191, 215
Deuteronomy, 33, 55,
diaphragm, 148
diazepam, 194

Dinah, 138
dirty, 138, 141
disability, 183
disciples, 185
discipline, 159
diseases, 66, 192, 199
disgrace, 67
dishonour, 141, 169
disinherited, 57
disobedience, 19, 64,
90, 92, 105, 219
Disorder, 195
disrepair, 174
distinction, 93
distinguish, 215
distress, 112
Divinity, 52, 83
DNA, 193
doctor, 76-77
dogs, 134, 208
dominion, 120
dowry, 128-129
dragon, 111
dreams, 65
drugs, 136, 193-194,
197-198, 200

E

Eden, 185
edification, 186
Edomites, 34

Index

Index

Index

Index

Index

Index